T0131625

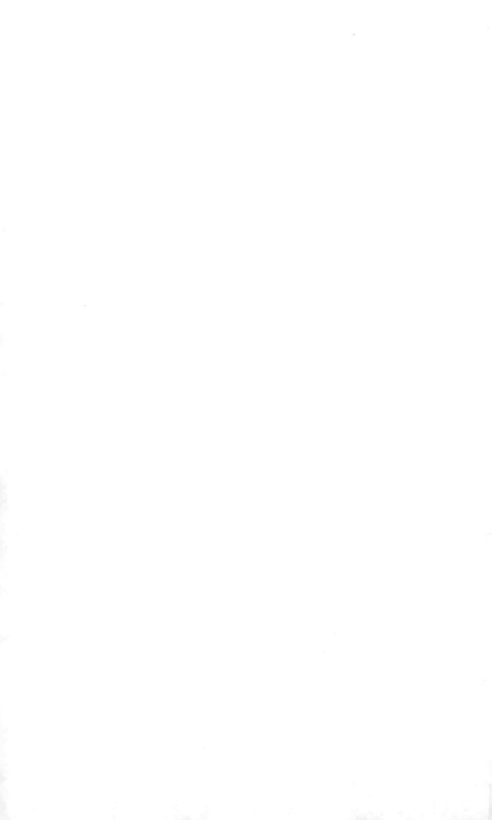

PRAISE

"This book is a call to action for physicians everywhere to embrace their natural leadership role and use the tools and resources available to them despite being mired by the various bureaucracies that often lead to burnout. The reader is given an excellent framework in starting the dialogue, sharing the strategies as well as the technologies that allow physicians to ask bigger questions and share their collective knowledge with one another. You are left with feeling there is no one better to shift the paradigm in healthcare than physicians and their dedicated teams."

— *Michael Leyson, MBA, Former Administrator Kaiser Permanente, Founder, The Leyson Report*

"A very accurate (tragically so) description of the problems faced by doctors and all healthcare professionals. Be prepared to be transported out of your comfort zone and projected into the 'uncomfortable truth.' As a friend and colleague, I was impressed by his ability to put into words the mix of feelings I have always had while working as an NHS doctor. A must-read for all the managers seeking to hear a different perspective from the inside with a vision that some of his proposed actions could become reality soon before it is too late."

— *Dr. Elisabetta Fabris, Consultant Acute Physician*

"This book takes me back to my eighteen-year-old self when being a doctor was all I ever wanted to do. The idea of using my skills and knowledge to make a real difference to patients' lives was my idealistic view of what my life would be like, how I would be valued, and what my purpose in life would be. I see it in my eighteen-year-old daughter as she waits for confirmation of an offer from a medical school—any medical school! Over the last twenty-nine years working in the NHS, although I still remember my initial purpose, it had been difficult, at times, not to feel disempowered, frustrated, and wonder whether it is all worth it—and I know I'm not alone.

Dr. Garbelli's excellent and original text is very timely, after a global pandemic, to give doctors the tools to cope with the daily frustrations of being a doctor and to rekindle their passion for medicine, thinking back to their eighteen-year-old selves. I highly recommend this book to allow young and not-so-young doctors to discover their true potential so that they can be their best and deliver the best possible care to their patients."

– Dr. Sarah Frankton, FRCP, PhD, Chief
Medical Officer, Consultant Physician

"As doctors, most of us become good at hiding our feelings and insecurities from others, including patients, their relatives, and our own nearest and dearest. Striving for the best outcome, we often ignore our personal (and family) frustrations while providing empathy to our patients. In this long-awaited doctor's manual, Dr. Pietro teaches us the importance of self-care and self-empowerment and how not to just survive but [also] thrive in a way only someone working at the coalface can!"

– Dr. Charles Li, Consultant Rheumatologist and Physician

"I am honored to have the privilege of reading this heartfelt account of experiences when working in medicine. One might believe that when training to be a doctor, rich rewards lie ahead in caring for and curing patients. While true, these will be tempered with often choppy and dangerous waters when trying to balance constant frustrations, particularly around bureaucracy and other irritations, when you are often made to feel that doing your best just isn't good enough. It is well documented that the ensuing effects on mental health are all too real and can have disastrous consequences on clinical staff. This book is to be commended for the depth of understanding and the sound suggestions and advice it offers."

– Jules Sleater, Associate Director Operations

"Much-needed book which is inspiring, positive, realistic, thorough, daring … and simply magnificent! Finally, the frustration of doctors dissected and precisely described. It gives back to us doctors the dignity of human beings who deserve to have a work environment that can allow us to be fulfilled, not only professionally, but also mentally and emotionally. I trust this will be a source of reflection for all the healthcare players, especially those who can make positive changes. I'm lacking in words to say how happy I am that finally I found a book where I can see my true reflection and that inspires me to face my frustrations head on. *Grazie*, Emanuele!"

— *Dr. Upinder Dial, Consultant Acute Physician*

"This book is refreshing. It is current and heartfeltly honest. I found each chapter captivating, easy to relate to what the author calls 'most beautiful profession in the world.' For a doctor like me, it was liberating to find thoughts and feeling discussed in the book that are very real and a testimony for many doctors: the passion of the calling, the daily struggles and frustrations, as well as the victories that keep us going. I found this book to be a positive motivating force, affirmation of why we want to address our frustrations, be good doctors, and remain in our profession as thought leaders. It is an empowering tool that drives the desire to make positive change in self and beyond, encourage us to have necessary conversations to 'heal the health of the system we work in' and nurture our minds. I recommend this as a must-read for every doctor and anyone interested in medicine, be it a medical stakeholder, a young person entertaining a career in medicine, or a service user. You are left with a feeling how powerful it would be for this material to be taught at medical school. I simply *love it*! Thank you, Dr. Pietro, for writing this much-needed book and for sharing your wisdom for the benefit of us all."

— *Dr. Anna Lukusa, General Practitioner*

"A fascinating book exploring the challenges doctors and other healthcare professionals face in today's healthcare system. Dr. Garbelli is clear, concise, and reflective, demonstrating a deep understanding of self-development, communication, and emotional well-being, while offering practical solutions. He also highlights the importance of these issues in relation to providing high-quality, patient-centered care. An extremely engaging read from start to finish."

— James Wood, Deputy General Manager, Medicine

"As a nurse and director of governance, I have seen my colleague nurses and doctors physically and mentally suffer in their very demanding roles. It's lovely to see that finally someone is writing about the struggles, and I can only highly praise Dr. Garbelli's openness when writing this book about the real struggles we face in healthcare. If we do not openly recognize these problems, we won't be able to tackle them, and they will stay hidden. Thank you for this amazing book, which hopefully will help many of our colleagues in their career paths."

— Ina Herridge, Director of Governance and Nurse

"As a cardiologist, I know the mechanics of the heart and how to perform a variety of cardiac procedures. However, when personal and work frustrations take over, they can impact our well-being, competence, patient care, and overall healthcare efficiency. Each chapter of this magnificent book makes you realize how the same devotion and commitment to growth and transformation is required at every level of the healthcare system. This God-sent and must-have guide creates a unique sublime fusion between subtle holism and modern conventional medical strategies as a brain booster to every doctor who is eager to transmute the frustrations into opportunities, create a nurturing medical environment, and be able to excel in our medical competence confidently."

— Dr. Todorche Stamenov, Cardiologist

THE
DOCTOR'S
VOICE

Empowering solutions to physicians' frustrations,
burnout, and healthcare inefficiencies

DR PIETRO EMANUELE GARBELLI

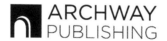

ARCHWAY
PUBLISHING

Archway Publishing books may be ordered through booksellers or by contacting:

Archway Publishing
1663 Liberty Drive
Bloomington, IN 47403
www.archwaypublishing.com
844-669-3957

Because of the dynamic nature of the Internet, any web addresses or links contained in this book may have changed since publication and may no longer be valid. The views expressed in this work are solely those of the author and do not necessarily reflect the views of the publisher, and the publisher hereby disclaims any responsibility for them.

Any people depicted in stock imagery provided by Getty Images are models, and such images are being used for illustrative purposes only. Certain stock imagery © Getty Images.

ISBN: 978-1-6657-3007-5 (sc)
ISBN: 978-1-6657-3006-8 (hc)
ISBN: 978-1-6657-3008-2 (e)

Library of Congress Control Number: 2022916950

Print information available on the last page.

Archway Publishing rev. date: 01/23/2023

DISCLAIMER

The advice and strategies found within this book may not be suitable for every situation. This work is sold to understand that neither the author nor the publisher is held responsible for the results accrued from this book's advice.

You may consider consulting with a professional (lawyer, health professional, financial advisor, etc.) for further details and future actions.

This book deals with many sensitive issues that doctors and other healthcare professionals and providers struggle with, and they often need more help than a book can offer. This book does not replace real therapy or qualified medical professionals. This book is only for informational and educational purposes and should not be considered therapy or any form of treatment.

The author cannot respond to specific questions or comments about personal situations, appropriate diagnosis or treatment, or otherwise provide any clinical opinions. If you think you need immediate assistance, call your local emergency number or the mental health crisis hotline listed in your local phone book's government pages.

The resources in this book are provided for informational purposes only. They are not there to replace the specialized training and professional judgement of a healthcare or mental health professionals.

The book is based on the experiences, opinions, and expertise of the author unless otherwise specified in the text or footnotes. If you are looking to use this book for research, please get in touch with the author and get the permissions required.

CONTENTS

FOREWORD

When I was asked to write a foreword for this book, I did so without hesitation.

I first met Pietro as a doctor in training in the United Kingdom recently arrived from Italy. He was seeking to develop his career and at the same time navigate the complex training environment that exists in the United Kingdom. His enthusiasm and willingness to learn and develop shone through even at that time. Reading this timely book, I am delighted that he has succeeded in becoming a consultant acute physician, but at what cost?

This book describes a personal journey from the child aspiring to be a doctor to an established consultant using "stories" and learning points to highlight some of the challenges doctors and indeed others working in health systems face. Some of the described events may appear difficult for some readers, but they will resonate with many. Each chapter explores potential frustrations, coping strategies, and solutions that could improve doctors' working lives and, as a result, improve care for patients at an individual or system level.

Dr. Pietro also displays a unique asset that other healthcare professionals could consider more often to seek help and self-understanding outside the system in which they are working; that for him encouraged reflection and a degree of calm. While, for some, this approach, to take time out or seek support directly, may not be possible, this book can provide useful pointers or help others in their personal and professional journeys as doctors.

His note about humor being used appropriately as a valued tool for coping and change is important. Individuals perform better when they don't dread their work but enjoy it and at times are able to have fun.

Each chapter of this book is a guide that helps doctors see they are not alone and that it is possible to navigate complex systems by asking questions of oneself, colleagues, and the wider system within a framework that works for them.

At the end of the day, the core message of the book makes us realize that people (staff) are the most valuable asset for any organization, and when they feel empowered and valued, they will provide the best care. High-performing teams have a common goal and deliver high-quality care. Thus, I highly recommend this book to all working in health and care, clinical and nonclinical.

Prof. Derek Bell, OBE
Professor of Acute Medicine Imperial College, London
Former President Royal College of Physicians, Edinburgh

INTRODUCTION

I have had the opportunity to coach, consult, train globally, and teach about the significance of values and the power of being authentic and purposeful, a key and rewarding component of Dr. Pietro Emanuele Garbelli's inspiring mission to Purposefully Transforming Healthcare®.

Deep in our minds and heart, we all have a purpose that we want to bring into this physical world. Why? Because, in addition to the emotional and psychological benefits, purpose can influence physical health. Having a strong sense of purpose can also help you be more focused, energized, and live longer. Now you can understand the benefits of doctors leading by example while being encouraged to be more empowered, healthy, and mindful. Being an empowered doctor far outweighs the risks of being frustrated, fearful, stressed, and vulnerable by living on the edge and uncertain about what the day ahead will bring into their life.

Over the years, I have been Dr. Pietro's coach and mentor. He has overcome many personal, relationship, and professional challenges that can leave any human being feeling burned-out, demotivated, depressed, on the verge of suicide, and considering leaving the profession altogether. One thing coaching and mentoring hundreds of doctors that I am sure is true is that the doctor's image is more of an idealized model that reflects people's aspirations rather than their experience.

Despite all the problems the COVID-19 pandemic brought to the NHS and government attention and the screen-time dedicated to them, the practice of medicine remains, for all practical purposes, invisible and underfunded.

While, on the one hand, the medical practice is continuously improving, the truth is it has not kept up with societal, regulator, and patients' rising expectations. If we were to use every orthodox and conventional measure, we would conclude that the NHS is better than it used to be. However, it is the well-measured truth that some things are much better than they were, but many other things are as good as people have been led to expect. The pandemic, the increased numbers of doctors leaving the profession, and those who commit suicide tell the darker lie— investment and access to care are essential only if the care itself adds value and makes a significant difference.

Until recently, what happened to patients once they reached the hospital or doctor of their choice has remained largely invisible. COVID-19 changed that daily. We were told how many people were infected, how many lives were lost, and what we all needed to do to contain the pandemic.

It also highlighted every problematic area of the healthcare system that could not cope because of long-term cuts in funds, training, and resources. Furthermore, doctors and all those working on the frontline were expected to be superhumans as they dealt with the aftermath of a healthcare system not prepared for a pandemic and the uncertainty it brought into our lives. The bar of what doctors were expected to do was raised. But too often the whole experience overwhelmed even the most vital doctors who cared for patients. The reason is the lack of values reflected in uncaring systems and growing bureaucratic processes is what leaves doctors and patients so powerless, frustrated, and frightened.

As someone who has spent thirty years leading and managing multimillion/billion technology-transformation programs, coached thousands of individuals from all professions, businesses from all market sectors, researched, studied, and learned various life disciplines, including engineering, business, technology, organizational and human behavior, self-empowerment, and psychology, one thing I realized is the hidden power of knowing our authentic values and how to align them with our daily actions and with the ones of the companies we work for. And how small and unexpected rewards can have disproportionate effects. We as human beings hold that satisfaction equals perception minus expectation.

The priceless yet straightforward values of empathy, tolerance, and trust—the graces of civilization—underpin the attributes of caring, honesty, good communication, and kindness. Those values struggle to survive in an underfunded, overmanaged, and under-led culture, one that fuels doctors' burnout, frustrations, and disappointments that negatively impact their personal, relational, and social lives; something that inspired Dr. Pietro to write this well-needed doctor's manual.

What Dr. Pietro is doing with this beautiful book is to address the frustrations that impact doctors and the healthcare system and start the conversations that need to happen to make known the source of such hindrances that are currently unknowable, like a cave that keeps its secret until the finest cave explorers explore it. In this book, Dr. Pietro realizes how those explorers are the doctors and nurses who resist the last thrusts of deconstruction.

We all know the importance of doctors' frustrations cannot be underestimated. Of course, there are many excellent, dedicated, caring, talented staff in the NHS who are its beating heart. I have had the pleasure to experience the caring and kindness offered by these people as a patient but also as a coach, educator, trainer, and partner who sees the impact the destruction of the environment and the culture in which doctors work has on their health, relationship, finances, and quality of life.

Since I started to coach Dr. Pietro, I intuitively knew that the journey we embarked on would eventually reveal a more significant role for him to play in Purposefully Transforming Healthcare®, with doctors playing a crucial role. At the beginning of our journey together, as his coaching partner, I helped him successfully overcome the pain of every frustration his doctor career created for him in his personal, family, and social life that you are about to read in this book.

It took a few years of coaching to get him to the point where he felt confident and empowered to write this book for you fellow doctors. In the five-day Vital Planning for Elevated Living Life and Business Mastery custom-made retreat at Zoëtry Paraiso de la Bonita, Riviera Maya, in Mexico, I coached Dr. Pietro for eight, at times ten, hours a day to help him clarify his vision, mission, and purpose. What came out of this advanced learning experience was a heavenly clear vision to purposefully transform healthcare.

I remember how we had tears in our eyes. We saw clearly how amazing implementing this vision would be for the NHS, the quality care patients receive, for doctors, for stakeholders, and for every healthcare provider in the world.

But then COVID-19 happened, the daily demands took over, and all we had worked together grounded to a halt. His doctor demands took over, and our focus became assisting him in successfully handling the personal and professional challenges that followed. When the travel restrictions were lifted and travel corridors were established, Dr. Pietro knew he needed a break to regain strength and continue what he started in Mexico. He booked another Vital Planning training, which took place in Cyprus. During this five-day intense coaching, I saw him go from not knowing he could write a book to creating the structure of the book you are now reading. He walked away feeling clear, confident, and content about writing and becoming a published author—a dream at the beginning of our journey he never thought he could achieve.

Yes, it takes commitment to drive such a purposeful vision into creation and make what once his mind perceived impossible become possible. It is what I love about Dr. Pietro. Despite all the challenges he faced, his commitment to writing this book, so other doctors could benefit from it, was unprecedented. It took some time for him to write, and we completed the final draft of this book a year down the line in another Vital Planning in January 2022 at Secrets The Vine in Cancún, Mexico. Seeing the joy in his eyes as he finished the first draft is what I know you as a reader will experience as you continue to read and uncover insights that will bring so much value to you as a doctor and to the environment you work in.

Throughout the book, Dr. Pietro brings to the readers' awareness the unintended consequences when a doctor's caring and kindness are divorced from delivering on targets. If the frustrations mentioned in each chapter that cause doctors not to perform at their peak continue unchallenged, then there is a fundamental problem that needs addressing now.

As someone who has assisted thousands of individuals and many companies addressing well-being, performance, productivity, profits and purpose-related issues, I believe that empowered doctors are the pulse of any healthcare provider's heart. Without investing in doctors' empowerment and continuous improvement and holding on to their authentic values, I know that there is a danger of becoming a demoralized profession, where nobody will tell the truth anymore about what is good and evil, right and wrong.

Drawing on the wisdom of his personal life experiences, the insights and research of case studies from his professional life, Dr. Pietro shows you how doctors' empowerment and inclusion is the foundation of making the process of Purposefully Transforming Healthcare® a successful and meaningful one that future generations will thank us for.

Dr. Pietro has managed to write an inspired book that takes you into an inside-out luminous reality of a doctor's life at every level of their existence. In every chapter, you will find ways to recover pathways to improve systems, processes, collaboration, support, technology, and a deep understanding of doctors' role in transforming the aging and underfunded healthcare system and meeting future demands. Dr. Pietro uses real-life doctor scenarios to encourage conversations that focus on finding meaningful solutions to ever-growing doctor and healthcare provider problems with great delicacy.

It is a compelling compilation of fascinating stories, personal experiences, and enthralling discoveries that awaken doctors' hidden potential, which healthcare providers can tap into as they meet the ever-increasing patient care demands of a future, where doctor artificial intelligence coexists with doctor human intelligence for the sole purpose of providing excellent quality care.

A common denominator for doctors is repeatedly experiencing frustrations that they bottle up, building pressure, and which at some point make them question the profession they chose to invest a lot of time, energy, and money in.

What many doctors tend to do at first about frustrations is to suck them up, keep quiet, and develop coping mechanisms to alleviate their pain. The current expectation is that, by using "healthy" coping mechanisms rather than "unhealthy" ones, doctors will be able to endure all the frustrations and stress provided by their jobs for the entirety of their working lives. But what Dr. Pietro is questioning in this book is, is this indeed possible? And are coping mechanisms labelled as "healthy" genuinely healthy?

Most biological, mechanical, and mathematical models include a point at which systems become saturated and stop being efficient or break. Then the question we must ask ourselves is, why do we expect doctors to defeat common physical laws and display superpowers absorbing and processing an unlimited amount of stress?

What triggers us, which we individually perceive as frustration, varies just as much as the strategies we develop as a response. Still, it is undeniable that there are common patterns that can be observed despite all this variability. Articles, editorials, surveys, and studies reporting that medical professionals struggle with various issues are widespread. If, like me, you coach and speak to doctors regularly, you'll come to understand how they usually are very vocal about their struggles, and you will be able to grasp the nuances of the problems which elude statistical data collection.

It is widely recognized that more and more doctors are self-reporting growing levels of dissatisfaction with their jobs, symptoms of burnout, and a range of mental health issues. Some end up reducing working hours, migrate to places around the world searching for better working conditions, and others take the route of changing the workplace, pursuing new careers, or retiring early. Various research shows how many doctors tragically take their lives at a significantly higher rate than other professions.

As the medical workforce continues to shrink for all these reasons, fewer doctors remain subject to increasing pressures in a never-ending vicious cycle. One cannot help but wonder, are the doctors, healthcare providers, and all those involved in healthcare asking the questions that can solve these ever-growing doctor, patient, and healthcare industry-wide issues?

Furthermore, doctors, in general, and the ones I have coached over the years, often forget to look at the effects of stress and frustrations on all areas of their lives: What about physical well-being and longevity besides the usual metrics on staff sickness levels? What about the impact on emotional well-being and long-term intellect besides the typical mental health diagnoses, burnout, and suicide metrics? How about the effects on the relationships with loved ones, their social lives, wealth, and spirituality? But do you think their partners, friends, families, and patients overlook the impact on every aspect of their lives? Doctors might be turning a blind eye to these effects, but how about their unconscious minds?

In the face of the COVID pandemic, the issue of healthcare staff well-being became a mandate and the number of initiatives multiplied. For some doctors, this has been a unique opportunity to experience, for the first time, practices, such as mindfulness, meditation, yoga, tai chi, journaling, coaching, mentoring, energy healing, etc.

Pietro is a doctor who has been committed to his self-growth and his coaching with me for the last six years. The transformations I have seen in him have made him an experienced doctor in self-development, familiar with and regularly practicing most of the above disciplines. Over the years, I have observed how he has regularly experienced vast amounts of stress and frustrations. Despite it all, he chose to empower himself to be the most excellent doctor he could be. Even before COVID, he was pretty underwhelmed (actually, enraged) by being offered these well-being modalities and resilience courses as the solution for doctors' troubles. While all the above methods have value in dealing with some of the stressors that lead to frustrations, they do not tackle the root cause of the problem.

A myopic view searches for solutions to help doctors cope with ever-rising challenges, such as increasing workload, increasing diagnostic complexity, time constraints, staffing shortage, rising expectations, increasing complaints and litigation, increasing bureaucracy and administrative tasks, quality improvement, risk management, education, training, the list goes on, but if you were given a choice between coping and thriving, would you even have to think about it? Do you, as a doctor, really want to set the bar so low that you accept survival as a standard expectation for a whole profession instead of aspiring the best?

Throughout the book, Dr. Pietro makes a case of what would be achievable if the energy you as a doctor currently use to develop and implement coping mechanisms were available for something else.

Each time I had to go to the hospital, I have often seen the pain and the fear in the eyes of other patients realizing they are about to be looked after by a struggling team of healthcare professionals. We know they are trying to do their best despite the challenges, but we also intuitively know when they are not at their best, at their peak performance. When our health is at stake, we realize it is priceless, and for the same reason, what we want is the best healthcare we can get.

Dr Pietro Emanuele Garbelli

I also know that those of you who choose to be doctors want to give your best as much as possible. Not being fully supported to do so all the time is a significant source of frustration and stress.

Not having control over your work and on how to improve your profession is another primary source of stress. Among unrealistic workloads, rigid guidelines, conflicting/overlapping deadlines, excessive regulatory burden, excessive bureaucracy, top-down imposed "improvement" activities, etc., your ability to have a say about what you do and express your uniqueness is remarkably restrained.

How many of you who work as doctors feel you are being asked to work more and more like a robot?

As the complexity of healthcare continues to grow, what is expected by doctors grows in parallel. It is time that we approach with critical and objective thinking all the support mechanisms and obstacles affecting doctors if we want to strike the balance right and keep a tidal wave of professional exodus and hindrances to performance abide.

Although we might sometimes feel as if we are drowning, there is still plenty we can do to avoid the ship sinking.

Drawing from personal experience, observations, and learning in personal reflection and coaching, what Dr. Pietro shares in this book are some solutions to common doctor problems that can help you be more empowered, energized, and effective. Those he chose to focus on in this book to start the conversations are

- identifying frustrations that lead to burnout;
- wide spectrum workload planning that leads to stress reduction;
- addressing the distrust that leads to poor priority management;
- preventing conflicts and creating a harmonious workplace;
- speaking in ways others listen;

- improving bidirectional information flow for greater efficiencies;
- playing an active role in using, maintaining, and shaping technology solutions;
- raising awareness of the need for comprehensive doctor protection;
- smarter ways of looking at doctor remuneration; and
- building a thriving culture through promoting the fulfilment of shared values.

Remember, many benefits come with pursuing a career in healthcare. As the field grows, new and exciting opportunities will emerge for healthcare workers. In the book, you will learn more about what puts many doctors off to remain in the profession that they invested years into and what can be done to encourage more doctors to stay at work. How to transform the mania for excessive paperwork and the setting of unrealistic targets that negatively impact doctors' well-being, interfere with providing good quality care and, in the NHS, eliminate a form of corruption much worse than the monetary kind.

Every chapter in this book, in one form or another, highlights how the entire system can be purposefully transformed by addressing the unintended consequences of doctors' frustrations. And if not addressed, the good doctor-patient relationship becomes unattainable, something medical care cannot function without.

In reading this book by Dr. Pietro, I trust you'll walk away with having a greater understanding of the fundamental challenges medicine and doctors face in the now and the future. Perhaps it will make your attempt to reconcile the inexcusable and ill-judged with influencing a "clever" healthcare strategy. You may even reach out to Dr. Pietro or us both to assist you in this journey, where Purposefully Transforming Healthcare® becomes that which sits at the heart of your healthcare organization.

Dr Pietro Emanuele Garbelli

Doctors' social and professional networks often overlap, which is why I hear in my coaching sessions with doctors that many doctors fear to say what they think. Dr. Pietro will challenge and inspire you to open up the needed dialogue for these two worlds to coexist beautifully without compromising the well-being of doctors, patients, and healthcare providers.

You also may use what Dr. Pietro shares to make a case of how providing doctors with a mechanism to put things right by speaking their minds and how you can develop them as healthcare thought leaders who purposefully transform your healthcare organization.

Whether we like it or not, evolution will ensure that cultural, technological, and structural change in healthcare will happen; it may well occur with purpose leading the way.

Before you continue reading this timeless book, let me leave you with a message worth adopting and sharing:

"Empower your doctors so they can be at the heart of the change that creates newfound empowered leaders of the NHS and healthcare systems around the world. Let them be the springboard of rediscovering lost values and creating innovative empowering solutions to take the healthcare system where doctors and everyone involved can thrive and strive for excellence in every aspect of quality care."

With love and wisdom,

Tony J. Selimi - Award-Winning Author, Speaker, and Transformational Life and Business Coach Specializing in Human Behavior, Purpose-Driven Authentic Leadership, and Maximizing Human Potential. Winner of the London SME Most Visionary Entrepreneur 2020 Award, Corporate Coaching and Recruitment Business Coach of the Year 2021 Award, Silver Winner of Literary Book Award 2021, and Maincreast Media Book Award 2021 for A Path to Wisdom, #Loneliness, and The Unfakeable Code®.

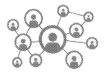

SHARING ME TO SERVE YOU

IF YOU PICKED UP THIS BOOK, THEN YOU MOST LIKELY REACHED A point in your career as a doctor where you can no longer stand feeling unheard. You probably have been questioning many aspects of your job, perhaps including whether to reduce your commitment or quit altogether. For sure, you are looking for solutions, just as we do for our patients. And if you are not a doctor, kudos to you for showing an interest. I promise this book has great value for you too.

Some of you may be also wondering who I am and why I have decided to write about/to frustrated doctors. The truth is by writing about doctors' frustrations, my aim is to also raise awareness about the frustrations of all professionals and not only within healthcare.

Work-related frustrations are so common that in many cultures, moaning about one's job is a common prop to initiate conversation with strangers, coworkers, and family members. For sure everybody has many reasons to be frustrated in their personal or professional field. If there ever were a "frustrated people's party", it would win any election as a landslide—and in many cases, it has!

I believe it's important to address doctors' frustrations because, if ignored, they have profound negative effects affecting not just doctors and everyone involved in healthcare, but also the very same people we are looking after: the patients. Something you will learn more about later in this book.

I chose to write about/to doctors because this is the area I have the most experience, subjectively and through talking with colleagues from different grades, specialties, and working in different countries. As you come to understand, the same principles and methodologies discussed in this book would likely apply to other healthcare professionals.

While it would be impossible to tackle every frustration we as doctors experience, my focus in this book is writing about solutions to common doctors' frustrations and unveil the positive consequences of doing so.

Let's say you made a note of the frustrations you experienced daily in your professional career over time, what number would you have reached by now? After a while, you may have noticed that most of those would be repetitions or only slight variations around the same issues. If you paid even more attention to what is happening to you throughout your working day, most likely you would still capture new ones as new experiences occur.

In my experience, we only share some types/sources of frustration with colleagues in the same workplace. Why? Because each of us experiences the world differently and has different expectations and unique sets of values (more on this later); therefore, our individual frustrations vary. Also considering differences in background, education, culture, beliefs, workplace, healthcare system, age, role, etc., one cannot help but wonder, how many frustrations do we collectively experience?

Changing jobs or workplaces is often perceived as a way to "leave behind" old frustrations, but soon enough, we encounter countless new ones. How to even start talking about such a huge topic is a hurdle on its own that many of us doctors need to overcome.

"How do you eat an elephant? One bite at a time."

My intentions are to share insights, instigate reflection, sparkle conversations, promote thinking "outside the box," and empower other doctors to be changemakers, so instead of cataloguing or systematizing frustrations in an analytical scientific way, I chose ten common sources of frustrations which have been recurrent themes in my own and my colleagues' experience as doctors. Those I focused on are what stimulated my desire for self-reflection, learning, and ultimately embarking on a personal growth journey, which I am inspired to share with you. I trust that what you will be reading throughout this book is what inspires you to look at your own frustrations differently.

First and foremost, I am dedicating this book to fellow doctors. However, what I am writing about will also speak to everyone working *in* healthcare, *with* healthcare, or *interested in* healthcare, such as managers, executives, policymakers, politicians, regulators, professional societies, insurers, suppliers, among others. As a way to start meaningful conversations and transform working relationships, please share it with everyone you believe should hear the messages it carries, be it your family/partner, your colleagues, your superiors, your employees, your managers, your trainees, other healthcare workers, etc.

I believe this book has the potential to improve and transform, not only the lives of doctors, but also many others, and by reading it, I hope it will reawaken within you the certainty that you can do so too.

As I trust that you, my reader, are another equally busy individual, I opted to keep this book concise and to get to the point fairly quickly in each chapter. Those of you who are more interested in hearing further on how the ideas shared can be conversation-starters, I invite you to reach out for further collaboration.

I also love to acknowledge and endorse the numerous teachers and mentors encountered throughout my life, and I will occasionally explicitly mention some of them in the text or footnotes. As this is meant to be a useful and pragmatic book for fellow doctors, and neither an academic bibliography nor my autobiography, my brevity is not a reflection of the gratitude and love I have for all of you who positively contributed to my growth and transformation.

How This Book Came to Life

Often it is at the worst times, when our lives are threatened, that we make a decision to do something about it. At the outbreak of the COVID-19 pandemic, as the news of the epicenter in Europe being in Northern Italy started to be shared, I was instantly alarmed that it would not have been long before it would have reached the United Kingdom. Fellow colleagues from Italy started reaching out and sharing all the information they had about the disease, the complications they started to observe, the protocols they had implemented to protect themselves from the virus, and the empirical treatments they started in the patients affected. At the same time, the instructions we received on how to handle the situation locally was confusing to many of us, our voices as professionals in our field were often ignored, and we were told to just follow orders.

Soon after being instructed to downgrade the protective personal equipment, I found myself ill with this new insidious virus, being forced to find creative ways to be tested at a time when staff testing was not even "set up." I ended up isolating myself at home, and only thanks to friends I had access to groceries and medications. I was encouraged to go back to work as soon as the fever subsided. Having been denied a further test to check whether I was still contagious (I continued to have a productive cough for another two weeks), I chose to wear a surgical mask to protect others. In doing so, many of us ended up being blamed for wearing masks in the hospital corridors and other public areas by people working in the hospital instructed by managers to discourage use of PPE outside clinical areas. The truth is no one was prepared to handle the complexities that the COVID pandemic brought upon our lives.

The frustrations I already had about my workplace and the profession exponentially multiplied in a matter of days; this was not anymore a matter of stress, but one that was putting my life and other people's lives at risk. I could not see a way out. I heard very similar stories from most colleagues I was in touch with. Days turned into weeks, weeks into months, and I was desperately seeking an escape where I could de-stress, find healthier ways to cope, and come back to work feeling more energized and clearer about what we as doctors can do to provide high-quality patient care while preserving our well-being.

Once the COVID turbulent waters calmed down, later in the summer, the government opened up Safe Travel Corridors. I booked a five-day Vital Planning Business and Life Mastery training in Cyprus with Tony J. Selimi, a globally renowned transformational life and business coach specializing in human behavior. At the beginning of my training, we addressed many of my doubts, fears, challenges, frustrations, and pains and made plans for the future. The truth is the desire to use all that pained me for assisting other doctors feeling equally angry, demotivated, and frustrated was built through years of investing in my personal and professional coaching and development with Tony and completing the Advanced Management Program on Health Innovation organized by the European Institute of Innovation and Technology.

Although an inspiring vision to Purposefully Transforming Healthcare® was born on another earlier Vital Planning with Tony in Mexico, what that meant in practice, I yet had to clarify. In each of the coaching and training sessions, I would bring a basket full of frustrations, issues, and problems. What would happen is I would walk away with learning more about myself, what is more important to me, what my authentic values are, and what my role in the bigger picture of life is. My perception back then was that I had not much value to give to others, that my ideas and insights had no worth, and that my only contribution to healthcare was my academic training and being good as a doctor in my clinical practice.

What Tony did for me, one can only describe as transformational work. He first asked me specific questions designed to extract all that was going on in my head. We wrote down all the doubts, desires, fears, frustrations, pains, and everything that was going on in my head. Then we started to categorize, organize, and prioritize all the information into clear topics that made perfect sense to me.

He used his unique book writing process to help me design every chapter of the book you are currently reading. I walked away being in awe of the transformation I experienced and what I was able to accomplish for you, fellow doctors.

Could have I written this book sooner? Yes. However, like you, I have been very busy dealing with patients affected by the virus and with the impact on an already extremely challenged healthcare system. I had to wait until my next holidays to dedicate time exclusively to writing and then reviewing the initial draft.

Undoubtedly, COVID brought plenty of new frustrations to our lives. Furthermore, while, on one hand, it temporarily allowed us to concentrate for a while purely on clinical work, temporarily pressing the "snooze" button on other duties, on the other hand, it unraveled even more most of the preexisting frustrations forcing us to continuously prioritize tasks and struggle with deadlines regarding nonclinical duties.

Despite several enthusiastic declarations that the pandemic would have accelerated many improvements in healthcare, two years down the line, we haven't seen much in terms of tangible advances affecting our professional lives.

May the topics shared in this book contribute toward having the necessary conversations and find the solutions required to transform and "heal" healthcare. May they become the necessary foundation upon which future changes and improvements can be safely and purposefully built upon.

Dr Pietro Emanuele Garbelli

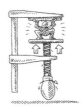

FRUSTRATIONS CAN EITHER MAKE OR BREAK YOU

BY THE TIME I TURNED EIGHTEEN, I WAS SERIOUSLY CONSIDERING medicine as my preferred career choice. It was so much so that if anyone asked me "What do you want to do in life?" my answer became invariably, "I want to be a doctor!"

It had taken me a lot of thinking and ruling out several other career options bit by bit. So you can imagine my mix of surprise, disappointment, and shock when I heard the following remark:

"If you want my advice, don't go to medical school. Being a doctor has become very difficult and frustrating nowadays. And as I don't expect things changing anytime soon, I would not wish that upon anyone. But"— as he noticed the uncomfortable expression building on my face—"if you have already made up your mind, then go ahead and become a *good* doctor. We always need those, and in the right circumstances, it is the most beautiful profession in the world!"

This was the *unsolicited* advice I was given by the doctor assessing my fitness for military service at age eighteen. He told me this as soon as he found out that I was considering applying to study medicine once graduating from high school. But by then, I had become used to hearing sentences like this from most of the doctors I encountered.

Not all of them tried to discourage me from studying medicine, but with few exceptions, most of them were visibly frustrated. And in some cases, they appeared disillusioned and bitter; the term *burnout* wasn't yet popular back then. As soon as they heard that I was contemplating becoming a doctor, they showed their interest, shared a piece of their mind, and often also openly shared some of their frustrations about the profession with a potential, future colleague.

In all honesty, back then, those words didn't really impact my decision. Trying to decide what to do with my life was my only concern. So I paid little attention to other people's professional frustrations, or at least I did not take those into account when weighing the pros and cons of different career choices. I assumed those frustrations were brought about by personal or local circumstances rather than a problem affecting the whole profession.

I've always listened to people's descriptions of lifelong vocations with a mix of envy and inadequacy. I remember playing the game *Operation* as a kid and being curious whenever visiting my pediatrician/family doctor's office, the biochemical analysis laboratory, or occasionally the hospital. But if you had asked me what I wanted to be when I grew up, I would have probably answered "an inventor," "a dancer," or "a musician" rather than "a doctor." The idea of studying medicine came to my mind much later because of a series of events.

When I was sixteen years old, on a Sunday morning, while I was in church with my family, I suddenly experienced a knife-like pain in my chest, like a stabbing, which lasted only a few seconds. I coughed a couple of times, then the pain stopped, leaving me puzzled about what just happened. Obviously, given the circumstances, my first thought was that God was sending me a signal. He was probably punishing me for being gay (not that I had done anything *about* it, quite the opposite). But the guilt I was living with, cleverly corroborated by the church, had made me see the world through shame-tainted glasses.

The following day, at high school, I realized something was wrong, during my physical education class. I could feel something hitting against the inner side of my chest wall each time I jumped. From my knowledge of biology, I was pretty convinced it must have been my lung bouncing inside my chest, but I had no idea why. I went to my family doctor the next day, and he organized an X-ray of my chest, which confirmed that my lung had partially deflated and it was floppily bouncing around inside my chest. I learned that the condition was named pneumothorax, and I was immediately held in the hospital and admitted to a surgical ward.

This was the first time I spent time in the hospital as an inpatient. I had a thick plastic tube inserted in my chest, connected to a big glass bottle half filled with water. I carried it around inside an old, rusty metal trolley with two wheels, one leg, and a long handle. I was told to be careful not to tip it over; otherwise, air would have leaked back into my chest, deflating the lung again.

But despite the wonky trolley and the long piping, I got so bored of staying in one room that I started wondering the whole hospital, particularly in the evenings. After dinner was served and all the visitors had left, the night shifts started. The squeaky and odd-looking apparatus I was dragging with me in the corridors attracted the attention of other wanderers and gave me a way to start many conversations. After several days, the air stopped escaping my lung, the drain stopped bubbling, and it was removed. And I was sent home.

Unfortunately, over the following few months, the same problem reoccurred twice. I ended up being admitted again, having more drains inserted, and I was transferred to a bigger hospital for an attempt to prevent further episodes by performing surgery. Between hospital admissions and outpatient appointments for scans and follow-ups, I ended up having an in-depth, first-hand experience of hospitals.

I was grateful to the nurses for taking great care of me. I was younger than the other patients, and I must have looked scared, so they often checked how I was feeling and encouraged me. They also gave me extra portions from the food trolley. I was skinny then, and since lots of the other patients were fasting, because of either being prepared for or recovering from surgery, there was always some extra food for me! In the evenings, when everything was quieter, I observed the night-shift nurses gathering to share some food and a chat. This often included a glass of wine and perhaps a cigarette and lots of coffee. *Oh, how things have changed!*

I remember thinking they had a nice social life, meeting a lot of people at work and having some opportunities to socialize with colleagues, compared to my lonely life as a nerdy student. Hospitals at night were an opportunity to meet new people. I remember escaping the wards and joining other patients in the garden for a chat and a sneaky pizza. *Hospital food has never been good anywhere I have been!* Since most patients who gathered into the garden were smokers, I even had a few puffs myself. I thought that, since my lung had already "given up" on me unexplainably, without me being a smoker, I might as well take the opportunity to try it and enjoy the company!

Besides being fascinated by the social aspects of hospital life, I was also intrigued by the technologies used: anesthetics, drains, sutures, casts, scanners, blood tests, miniaturized video cameras, surgical instruments, etc. At the same time, I was often disappointed by the apparent lack of empathy of many doctors I interacted with, and also by the scarcity of opportunities to enquire about the cause of my disease, how to prevent further episodes, and how it would have impacted my future.

I started thinking, in some cases, *it seems they don't care, I wonder if they are always like this, I would have said that differently*, and occasionally, even *I would be better at it!*

Imagining how I would/could have *been* in the same situation *on the other side of the fence* is one of the things I attribute my vocation to.

By the time I was eighteen, medicine was among the top choices I was considering for my future studies. But it took me a long time to decide. Having had an eclectic interest in many studies and topics and having to suddenly choose just *one* for the rest of my life felt daunting. I spent a long time weighing the pros and cons of different university courses then narrowed down the options to a dozen. I kept an open mind about the other options until I received the results of the entry test for medical school. Being in the top ten, among thousands of applicants, felt like a sign that I was on the right path. So I trusted that feeling and enrolled in medical school with conviction.

Of course, ending up in a hospital as a patient wasn't the only factor that brought me to choose medicine. I always had an interest in biology, science, and technology. Plus, I shared some humanitarian traits with my mother, who was a social worker. Helping others appeared a worthy thing to do for a living, and it was something I would not get bored of easily too.

My religious upbringing definitely played a role too. At a time, when I was still fighting against my sexual orientation and being surrounded by societal homophobia, bullying, and religious prejudice, I thought helping others for a living would have made me more socially acceptable in the eyes of others *and God* and allow me to have a *less horrible* life.[1] Those were the times when no positive gay role models were in sight. Judging by the people I was surrounded by, the media, and the church, the only available alternatives would have been to be laughed at and continuously discriminated against, live in the shadows and hide *or be ordained*, be beaten up and maybe killed, or die of AIDS alone, rejected by family and society.

---

[1] Internalized homophobia accounts for many gay men overachieving in studies and careers to compensate for low self-worth and fear for the future as we read for example in *The Velvet Rage: Overcoming the Pain of Growing Up Gay in a Straight Man's World* by Alan Downs.

But let's fast-forward in medical school. After the first three years, dedicated to the exact and reassuring world of basic sciences, I was then introduced to the hospital environment for the following three years. The rigors and exactness of science were replaced by the uncertainties of clinical medicine. For example, we learned in how many surprisingly different ways diseases might present themselves and how to collect clues and recognize them. Other notable differences compared to the previous years were that we started receiving lectures by doctors rather than just university professors and lecturers, and we spent time in rotation in all hospital departments learning about diagnostics and various aspects of clinical medicine, where our tutors were doctors.

I believe our tutors didn't necessarily have any extra time protected from clinical duties to look after us students; it was just expected of them as common duty of those working in a teaching hospital and among other challenges they must have faced, occasionally their frustration was palpable, and it wasn't always the best experience for us students. Nevertheless, I am now very grateful for all the efforts and dedication they put into transmitting their knowledge and skills to us, and I am also grateful for not having given up on finishing my studies despite again being surrounded by so much frustration among my future colleagues.

During the last few years at university, the clinical commitments progressively increased, eventually spending plenty of time as intern medical students on a ward of our choice and carrying out research for the final dissertation. Besides learning about clinical medicine, I learned about hospitals as a workplace; my idealized expectations of fairness, equanimity, solidarity, etc., were soon replaced by firsthand experience of unfairness and power games: nepotism, exploitation, corruption. Thanks to my family's upbringing, I detested corruption, nepotism, favoritism, and servility, and I started wondering if I could ever *fit in*. Refusing certain compromises also sometimes meant taking difficult decisions which progressively led me far away from home.

For example, to start postgraduate studies immediately after graduating from university, I had to move away from my native region, but this also became an opportunity to start living independently, acquire adult life skills, make new friends, have an initial experience as a "migrant," and have fun.

During my specialty studies, I encountered good mentors and started friendships that last to these days. Occasionally, I had to stand up for myself and keep the morale up despite the challenges and despite witnessing much suffering, not only among patients, but also among fellow doctors of all grades.

Once completed my specialty studies, I hit a first life crisis; after having encountered so many frustrated, disheartened, burned-out doctors throughout my training, my self-preservation instinct "kicked in" very strongly when I came to the point of deciding about my future professional life. For a while, all I could think of was *I do not want to become like them!*

I also knew that in a corrupt environment, I would have suffered too much trying to grasp some half-decent career opportunities without compromising too much on my principles.

As I could afford being without a job for a while, and as all I was certain about at the time was what I *did not want* but struggled to be in touch with knowing what I really wanted to do with my life, I took some time off to reflect and do some soul-searching. I asked myself a lot of uncomfortable questions, researched and pondered over a lot of alternatives, until I eventually decided that migrating to a country with fairer career opportunities was going to give me the best chances.

Fast-forward to the present and I often find myself saying about migrating, "I assumed the grass was greener on the other side, but in reality, it's just a different hue of s**t!". What I really mean is *migrating wasn't the solution.*

By all means, I had a good career, learned a lot, flourished as a doctor, became a good teacher, started and/or got involved in many projects, helped over fifty thousand patients, and worked with great colleagues, but despite all these, I found myself so often being the very thing I so much wanted to avoid: another frustrated doctor.

Having been a patient myself several times, also later in life, and having gone through good and bad experiences, i.e., having experienced and observed positive and negative role models as the receiver, contributed profoundly to shaping my professional values, behavior, and ethos. At the beginning of my career, I had high expectations about myself: I set out with the intention of being a great doctor; to be compassionate, caring, knowledgeable.

As I found out later, holding up to these high standards all the time hasn't always been easy or possible; the difficulties, challenges, restraints, and idiosyncrasies of various workplaces, bit by bit, unconsciously molded and shaped my behavior until I ended up sometimes catching myself being grumpy, rushed, frustrated, overwhelmed, angry, impatient, pretty much everything I had intended to avoid becoming.

Was it only a matter of unrealistic expectations? Partially yes, a one-sided expectation equals chasing a dream, an illusion. But it was also an eye-opener that forced me to look inside and around me to understand why I, like so many of my former and contemporary colleagues, ended up experiencing symptoms of professional burnout.

A second life crisis hit me a few years back, when, at some point, I was seriously contemplating leaving the medical profession altogether and dedicating my life to doing something completely different in hope to find some peace and be surrounded only by harmony and love. I talked about it, fantasized about it, but I never really took action; something was blocking me, but I didn't know what. I felt lost. I feared throwing away all the years and sacrifices I had made to master a profession that was causing me recurrent pain. I still enjoyed many aspects of it, such as caring for the patients, making a diagnosis, working with nice colleagues, learning something new, teaching younger colleagues, but there were so many things I was forced to do or endure that I just hated. Was it really worth it?

Exactly at that time, I was introduced to life and business coach Tony J. Selimi and was invited to talk to him about my plans about an alternative career; after we met for coffee and an initial consultation, I started working with him and never stopped. I quickly realized that deep down, I did not authentically want to quit medicine. I still loved my profession. I was struggling with some aspects of the *environment*, the way healthcare organizations and hospitals were *forcing* us doctors to work.

Patiently and with dedication, I embarked in a long introspective and evolutionary journey, overcoming many challenges, learning not only about myself but also about human behavior in general, and slowly transforming my way of being. I learned how, by changing my perceptions, I could turn all the frustrations into an unlimited source for empowerment, making me a more confident and energized doctor, ready to take on the next challenge.

I kept working intensively with Tony, brainstorming and organizing the many ideas I had been having about improving the working environment for doctors, transforming hospitals and healthcare in general. Often we would address the many things that continued to trigger my anger and frustration. Having an inquisitive and introspective nature and having invested a lot over the years on personal development, I have observed in myself and others the pervasive slow and progressive negative effects of accumulated frustrations.

Having overcome some challenges and learned something in the process, I couldn't wait to share these learnings and insights which can support you as a doctor in similar situations. Furthermore, it can be a great way for gaining a different perspective for those with decisional powers who want to have granular insight and useful tools for creating a thriving working environment.

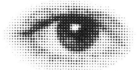

STOP IGNORING, START NOTICING

"Doctor, when I press here, it hurts. What should I do?"
"Stop pressing!"

I FIND THIS POPULAR MEDICAL JOKE QUITE CLEVER AS IT CAN BE interpreted in different ways; one of which is that the cause and perhaps the solution may be obvious and right under our eyes if we just *connect the dots*. I could not help but wonder if it can teach us something about the root causes of some of the most relevant emergencies affecting the medical profession nowadays: frequent workplace changes, hours reduction, early retirement, career dropout, migration, burnout, mental health issues, and suicide.

We are used at looking at these problems mostly in isolation, and this definitely has a purpose; for example, once a certain diagnosis has occurred, doctors may definitely need targeted support and sometimes treatment. But at the same time, I believe it is important we try to understand what these issues have in common, why it appears that their respective rates are slowly increasing over time, and what can be done to prevent these from occurring. As always, prevention would be better than treatment!

If these life events were not already worrying or tragic enough on their own, an additional concern for the profession, which increases the urgency for finding solutions, is the fact that what all these have in common is a progressive erosion of the workforce, while at the same time, the amount of work to be done slowly increases (because of an aging population, increasing comorbidity burden, increased diagnostic accuracy, etc.), resulting in a growing mismatch between workload and workforce. In other words, fewer doctors are left to deal with more work, and it is obviously not sustainable.

Two tip-of-the-iceberg issues mentioned above stand out from the others for their tragic nature and complexity; doctors can, like any other human being, suffer with mental health issues or commit suicide for reasons completely unrelated to their profession. Nevertheless, there must be reasons why the rates of these problems are higher among doctors compared to other professions and the general population.

If we leave suicide and mental health issues aside, another thing all these problems have in common is they are all symptoms of *dis*ease with or related to the medical profession; there is something making doctors fall out of love with the profession and/or their jobs years after the initial call/vocation, and the same might play a role in burnout too.

Having experienced some of the problems listed above myself, having observed them in many colleagues and trainees over the years, and having read a fair amount about these issues in specialized and general press, articles, studies, and books, my curious mind started inquiring and connecting some dots.

If you ask colleagues why they have decided to change workplace, go part time, retire early, or go all the way to migrate to another country to practice medicine or leave the medical profession altogether, they will often list many problems encountered that they perceived insurmountable until they reached a breaking point when they said to themselves, "Enough is enough!" and started looking for an alternative.

Admittedly, employers are meant to collect some data about this, for example, carrying out exit interviews when people leave a job; but often this is done badly or not at all and sometimes is delegated to using rigid questionnaires which do not give an opportunity to express the real reasons for such a decision. As a result, our employers might be blind to the real reasons why doctors are leaving and completely miss an opportunity to retain more doctors in the profession.

The truth is a lot more can be done before reaching the breaking point.

As doctors, many of us are used to moan about the problems we encounter at work and that frustrate us. We moan about them with our colleagues at work and sometimes outside work, with our partners and families, with our friends; even the most reserved, shy, and wise of us will have a good old moaning from time to time, just to "let the steam off" before going back to dealing with the same frustrating things. Moaning definitely has a function similar to the valve on a pressure cooker, letting some steam off (i.e., verbalizing stress) to prevent the pressure (stress) from rising to unsafe levels. But are we truly designed to function like pressure cookers, or does this valve sometimes fail to keep the pressure within safe levels?

Much has been written about stress and the effects that "bad" (i.e., persistent, repeated, avoidable) stress has on our minds, bodies, and on a larger scale, organizations, society, countries, etc. Some of the difficulties when studying stress are the subjectivity of what is perceived as stressful and the lack of an accurate tool to measure stress; for this lack of objectivity, we often fail to assess, acknowledge, and address stress in workplaces. We almost inevitably leave it to the individual to self-assess stress levels and self-manage stress-reduction strategies, but we rarely look at the causes of stress.

But what if there was another way?

When we moan about things that frustrate us, aren't we ultimately talking about things that trigger stress? And when those frustrations are experienced repeatedly, isn't that actual persistent stress? And when we moan about the things that frustrate us that nobody ever changes, haven't we just identified causes of persistent stress that could be changed?

Why not use frustrations as a tool to measure stress and identify and address its root causes?

My science-trained mind expects some partial objections at this point, so let me expand. Of course, we *could* conduct studies to measure the impact of stress-reduction on the various issues affecting us doctors using the solutions for capturing, reducing, and eliminating frustrations discussed throughout this book and see which issues may have a linear correlation and which ones might respond less because of multifactorial influences.

I estimate such a study would need to last at least five to ten years. However, I don't think we have the luxury of being able to wait so long for the results before implementing solutions to stop a tsunami of problems facing our profession just for the sake of being scientifically sound.

It is widely accepted that a randomized clinical trial to investigate whether using parachutes prevent deaths would be unethical and unnecessary. The same applies to studying whether administering oxygen to people with dangerously low oxygen saturation prevents immediate death; there are many cases in several fields where solutions have been implemented without awaiting the results of lengthy trials.

Moreover, how many doctors would even agree to be in the control group where the stress levels and frustrations remain unchanged for years?

So what can we do instead?

We can choose to see *opportunities* for learning, business, or whatever else or see *problems*. Which one we chose will determine the outcome. So why not choose to train our minds to see *opportunities for solutions* where we previously saw frustrations?

In other words, we can continue to ignore, or we can start noticing *frustrations as vehicles of information* regarding the most common sources of doctors' stress, specifically in our workplaces.

Instead of discounting moaning as just something we do with peers to feel temporarily better, or something others offload upon us which sometimes makes us feel temporarily worse, we could start listening, collecting the information, noticing patterns, analyzing, finding solutions to the problems identified, and eventually, implementing them.

Talking directly to doctors, asking questions and listening, conducting interviews, is always a great way to gather information about a workplace. Some may find it, at first, unscientific and might even label parts of it as "gossip," but if you pay attention, you will notice that it's used by many disciplines, anthropology, for example, and ultimately, by ourselves, when we collect history from patients. Of course, when it comes to big numbers of doctors, there is a need to design alternative methods to collect information.

Questionnaires and surveys are often used for this purpose, but they also have limitations; for example, a low response rate, the fact that they are a passive exercise (you are invited to respond), or the fact that the questions are predesigned, and you will only find out what you thought asking about. But what about those questions you never thought of asking?

The use of closed questions and prewritten answers not only limits the granularity but also the accuracy of the information collected; has anyone ever completed an entire questionnaire without being able to find "their" answer to some of the questions and being forced to choose something quite inauthentic just to move forward?

On the contrary, the use of open questions leads to the problem of requiring processing, interpretation, systematization, and ad hoc analysis. In small surveys, this can be done manually, and it usually provides valuable information, but on bigger scales, it has rarely been feasible until recently.

The use of applications on smartphones has greatly increased our interaction with technology, and the possibility of real-time communication has expanded our ability to collect data. Wearable technology is also increasingly popular. When it comes to data analysis and interpretation, another type of technology is required to go beyond the limited amount of information we can process as human beings.

With the advent of artificial intelligence and machine learning, new possibilities for analyzing data are being designed in a very rapidly evolving landscape. When it comes to imagining the applications for new technologies, our imagination is more often the real limit.

What if technology could analyze doctors' conversations, written or vocal, identify and communicate to us, and maybe our employer, our common frustrations? What if technology could pick up our frustration, anger, and stress level and help identify the contributing factors? What if technology were able to monitor these continuously throughout the day? What if the information were used, not only in solving issues and designing systems, but also instantly as correction in feedback loops?

For example, what if our computer, or whatever other piece of technology, was able to know that it is irritating us as doctors and adapt its 'behavior' and functions instantly?

I know that this opens lots of questions about privacy, data protection, how much we are comfortable to share information about our emotions, thoughts, and private lives, and how comfortable we are with a machine being able to measure how we feel, etc. In a dystopic view of how the future could look like, all these things could, of course, be used against us, but at the same time, in an optimistic and futuristic view, they could exponentially increase our well-being, productivity, comfort, efficiency, support us in accessing, analyzing, and interpreting data.

In my opinion, as these technologies are being developed whether we like it or not, we might as well *be in the driving seat*, guiding and influencing the design in a way that is supporting us doctors and making sure we identify and address possible problems that could arise.

As the current technology, mostly not designed by or with the help of doctors, is often a major source of frustrations, as you know and as you'll read in another chapter, having a chance to shape the technology that we are going to use in the future is an opportunity not to be missed! It is why I believe empowering doctors is a crucial step in this process of designing and influencing the technological future of healthcare.

The question also becomes, what else can we do in the meantime with the existing technology and within our reach?

In the following chapters, I write about some common frustrating problems I repeatedly encountered and possible solutions, starting from those which are achievable and in our hands. A common feeling I have experienced and observed time and time again is *disempowerment*: perceiving that we have no control over any of the problems affecting us, believing that the solutions depend on remote higher powers we cannot control or even influence, essentially feeling stuck and powerless.

But as you will read, our perceptions are often clouded or partial, and we have access to many alternatives. I trust that doctor empowerment, feeling that you can regain control of aspects of your professional lives, is going to help us going a long way. In fact, many other solutions, the ones we usually focus on, depend on decisions beyond our immediate sphere of influence; this is why I have spent some time suggesting not only these changes to those readers with decisional powers but also how to keep developing communication skills that can better support us in becoming efficient influencers and advocates for the changes we so desperately and urgently need.

In summary,

- Ignoring frustrations is what builds unnecessary stress.
- Despite all the current efforts, the rates of problems affecting doctors are rising.
- Moaning about frustrations doesn't solve them.
- The spectrum of problems affecting doctors have common causes.
- The models and solutions designed to address these problems are failing to show promised results.
- Prolonged stress is what leads many of us doctors to feel dissatisfied, search for ways out, develop mental health issues, drop out of the profession, and unfortunately, growing suicide rates.
- To empower doctors is to interrupt the progression of frustrations.

Before you move to the next chapter, let me leave you with a message worth spreading:

Empowered doctors are catalysts for purposeful healthcare transformation.

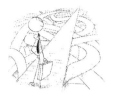

GOODBYE, CRISIS; HELLO, PLANNING

Are you familiar with the famous TV series *Star Trek*? In each episode, at some point, there is a threat that affects the spaceship and all its crew. The response is the activation of the red alert, which means "all crew must report to duty stations."

It certainly contributed to holding and heightening our attention as viewers. It satisfied our appetite for adventure, danger, excitement, creativity, uncertainty, and curiosity. The reason being each episode was focused on one crisis and the solution to the threat. This is what made it so addictive, fun, and successful.

Now imagine what would have happened if the writers of this epic series introduced crisis after crisis happening in just one episode. Would hearing red alerts every few minutes, without ever getting to the solution of the first red alert, keep you engaged, focused, and curious? Most likely you would lose your attention and interest within the first half hour. Why? Because our reaction to repeated sounds of danger would eventually change to annoyance, and besides feeling sorry for the poor spaceship crew, we would have soon changed the channel, and the series would have eventually been cancelled.

The situation isn't much dissimilar with us doctors working in many modern acute hospitals; as the influx of patients to the emergency services cannot be controlled,[2] fluctuations in the number of patients mean that on some days, the demand (i.e., the number of patients simultaneously requiring a service) exceeds the capacity (e.g., the number of beds available to admit patients), and alerts are sent throughout the organization to gather help. And if that help is not there because of lack of or limited resources, many doctors end up feeling overwhelmed, and if that continues over prolonged time, they will look for alternative jobs, just like the viewers of the alternative version of *Star Trek* would change channel.

It all sounds logical in theory, but let's dig a little deeper.

Long-term healthcare budget cuts have translated, at first, in closure of smaller hospitals, then into merging of hospitals into bigger trusts, sharing supporting services, outsourcing of most services to external companies, and eventually in closure of wards and reduction in hospital beds and staffing.

The underlying publicly declared intention was to promote efficiency, stimulate productivity, and promote alternative ways to provide healthcare that do not require admission to a hospital. While we can all subscribe to these targets (who doesn't want a flexible healthcare system capable to diversify its offering and deliver healthcare in ways that are less disruptive of personal life?), it doesn't take a Nobel Prize winner to figure out that productivity and efficiency applied to the part of healthcare delivered to inpatients cannot continue to increase indefinitely. The main limiting factor being the speed at which human bodies heal (unless of course we are aboard the *Enterprise* spaceship with instant-healing technology).

Inevitably, a point will be reached when the supply will be inadequate to address the demand. Moreover, this model fails to take into account that the demand itself for healthcare has been steadily increasing brought about by combinations of factors, such as increase in population, aging, lack of investment in prevention,

---

[2] Except for rare circumstances when ambulance emergencies can be temporarily diverted toward other hospitals

lifestyle, deprivation, side effects from treatments, and accumulation of diseases in clusters (comorbidities).

Days when hospitals struggled to provide care used to be a rare exception and unpredictable (apart from the effect of public holidays; see below), and sending an SOS across the organization to gather some help was a rare event, but over the last few years, the struggle has become more and more pervasive up to being a nearly daily occurrence in some organizations.

Because of the annual surge in infective illnesses in cold weather, we used to work extra hard over the winter months and struggle to accommodate demand on some days, while the relatively lighter summer months allowed us to dedicate more time to administrative and managerial tasks and allowed staff to go on holidays without impacting on healthcare delivery. Over the last few years, as a result of increase in demand and reduction in capacity, there has been no perceptible decrease in activity over the summer months with hospitals working nearly all-year-round at full capacity or over capacity.

Similar to the *Enterprise* spaceship in the *Star Trek* TV series, hospitals have adopted various ways to alert personnel of the impending danger, summon them, asking to drop all (but essential) activities to deal with the peril. What used to be an occasional *call to arms* has become a nearly daily cry for help, but what is the real effect of doing this?

Apart from the obvious risk to desensitize the response over time, as in the famous fable "The Boy Who Cried Wolf" by Aesop, and of excessive stress and burden to those constantly summoned to action without any downtime, the crude reality of many hospitals is that there are no "reserve doctors" available to jump into action; they will have to sacrifice something to do something else. Typically, they might be asked to drop every activity that is not directly patient-facing; this includes not just administrative, educational, and managerial tasks, but occasionally also acknowledgment of results, dictating and checking letters, etc.

Also, typically, when these alerts keep sounding nearly every day, it becomes difficult for the organization to think about alleviating doctors' workload, reducing the expectations, or discounting some lower-priority activities; at the most, they will sometimes move certain deadlines further. Even during the COVID pandemic waves, most of the activities cancelled to free up more clinical time during the peaks—such as responding to complaints, investigating minor and moderate risks and incidents, organizing appraisals, mandatory training, and continuous professional education—were still waiting for us as doctors to catch up with at the end, together with a huge backlog of clinical activity put on hold, such as outpatient clinics, investigations, and procedures.

Can you imagine what would happen to the *Enterprise* spaceship if its crew faced continuous red alerts being unable to complete their routine daily jobs? Eventually, it would become a shipwreck!

So what could be done differently?

If we look at nature and technology, we cannot help but notice that most systems are built with a *buffer* system to deal with fluctuations. For example, our bodies efficiently deal with variations in the type and amount of foods and liquids we ingest every, day maintaining relatively constant internal conditions, a process known as homeostasis. Several buffer mechanisms allow our bodies to maintain a relatively constant pH of the blood, despite ingesting lemon juice and vinegar one moment and bicarbonate or anti-acid remedy on other occasions.

Similarly, many systems conceived by engineers are designed to deal with a range of input larger or smaller than what is normally experienced during normal working conditions; for example, metals forming an airplane's wing or the structure of a bridge can occasionally absorb stronger forces and vibrations without breaking.

Another example of a buffer we use every day allows us nowadays to stream TV programs and webinars and make video calls without interruptions, invisibly dealing with an uneven delivery of chunks of information over the Internet.

So why don't we have buffers in hospitals?

A minor part of it depends on practical limitations; for example, when redesigning services in an existing hospital, we might have to adapt to an already-existing physical structure that doesn't allow expansion. That's how we often end up, for example, with waiting rooms too small for the number of patients or too few clinic rooms.

But when it comes to staffing levels, a culture of maximizing efficiency, if not careful, can hit us as a double-edged sword. The popular perception is that we are used to glorify being busy, sometimes describing our actions even as heroic. But then, when doctors ask for increased staffing levels, they are often faced with questions, such as "What will these doctors do for the rest of the day?" or negative answers, such as "I cannot justify X number of doctors/nurses in a department that only sees Y patients per day."

Unfortunately, we forget that efficiency is most needed in times of crisis to deal with a surge swiftly and go back to "business as usual" rapidly without the negative effects of the crisis rippling through the system for too long.

There are lessons we can learn from the military corps. They always have reserve soldiers ready to get into action whenever needed; having such reserve doctors in healthcare would allow doctors to face efficiently repeated surges of demand without accumulating significant backlogs. And that is something worth considering. In some countries, reserve/"floating" doctors and nurses are a reality.

A few years ago, having just redesigned and opened a service in a new area of a hospital, some managers visiting the service only a few days after it had reopened commented negatively about how empty the waiting room looked, "Like a shipwreck."

That comment made me reflect while it was true that the service had not reached full potential yet, I realized that a full waiting room is a sign of *inefficiency* and no way a measure for a successful launch. The truth is, with effective planning of appointments and processing, the waiting room, i.e., the buffer in the system, never overfills.

It is wise to design effective systems in a way that have some spare capacity to absorb fluctuations in the input without a decrease in overall performance.

What would having a buffer mean for doctors working in hospitals?

For example, having departments that are big enough to accommodate everyone at the peak of activity; having enough doctors and nurses that, on a "normal" day, don't have to rush at full speed, with clinics not completely booked or overbooked and wards not completely full, so that they can look after a few extra patients promptly when needed. It may also mean staff being allocated some extra nonclinical duties, beyond the bare minimum necessary to fulfil the organizational and professional requirements, who may be occasionally called back to clinical work in case of unplanned need.

While most professional contracts and job plans include protected time for such activities, in real-life scenarios and in a climate of continuous crisis, it is rare for doctors to be given "protected" time, and the amount of administrative work takes up all the time available, leaving very little or no time for anything else. As professionals in our field of work are required to (and interested in) continuously keep up to date and expand and refine their skills, struggling to do anything else but maximum-speed direct clinical care when at work is another big source of frustration.

In any decision-making, it is wise to look at both sides.

Having more doctors equals more salaries, more operational responsibilities, bigger space, etc., which is probably one of the main downsides from a managerial point of view. But are there other hidden advantages that may be beneficial to include in the cost-benefit analysis?

It is widely known that people who are constantly squeezed too hard become much less efficient at their jobs. Not only they are slower and at risk of making errors, with obvious repercussions not only affecting them individually but also the reputation and finances of the organization, but they will also have more sickness absences. Their loyalty to the organization will greatly decrease, and they will be much less keen to make any extra effort to help the organization in times of need. Some end up becoming even more demanding in terms of retribution (in other words, "If they want to make my life hell, they'd better pay me well for it!"), ultimately cancelling any perceived advantage of paying fewer salaries. The same applies to us doctors. By having more doctors, we can effectively use their "spare" time to focus on improvement work, thus increasing efficiency and also reducing waste.[3]

A general misconception is that doctors would inevitably take advantage of too much freedom at less busy times. However, we must not overlook the ongoing demands that leave many of us doctors with little down time to rest. As doctors, our primary drive is to provide excellent patient care; thus, it is for us doctors to use downtime to engage in activities that enhance our productivity, the service we work in, contribute to research, engage in other activities that interest us, grow our skills, and pursue our personal callings in life.

Wanting to improve oneself and continuously grow is deeply ingrained in our nature; doctors are no exception. Although some of us may express this in different ways, in general, as healthcare professionals, we have in common a desire to deliver high-quality care. However, as human beings, we all have a very unique set of priority values. By values, I mean the underlying drivers of our own

---

[3] Waste of time, resources, processes, money, etc.

actions, i.e., what is important for us and what we invest time and resources in.[4] As a result of having unique sets of values, it is essential to offer a selection of activities in our nonclinical time; one size does *not* fit all!

Let's look at other possible ways hospitals can fail to match demand and capacity.

A recurrent theme that can be observed across hospitals is poor advance planning around predictable events. I am not talking about the sophisticated predictions in surges of certain diseases by statistical models, such as what we have seen with COVID-19, but simply preparing for recurrent events, such as festivities, rotation of academic staff, seasonal sickness surges, maternity and paternity leave, etc.

Many of you doctors reading this book may empathize with the struggles to find last-minute solutions to problems that recur predictably every year, such as ensuring safe staffing levels during the Christmas period. The only variable is the number of days affected each year, but the approach on how to address the problem can remain the same. Unfortunately, we often find ourselves having to improvise the solution because of not retaining staff who already know how to do it and because we rarely write "how to" guides or find the time to read them when they exist.

In any case, these two approaches are not the same; retention of good employees (*know how*) by increasing job satisfaction cannot be substituted by bureaucracy (manuals, instructions, guidelines, etc.). Successful multinational companies know this and over the years, have shifted their attention toward looking better after their employees. Hospitals have been encouraged to do so too. Multiple staff well-being initiatives have been launched as a response to the COVID pandemic; some of which failed to reach the desired effect or to be available to the intended users, such as yoga classes at the

---

[4] See *The Values Factor* by Dr. John Demartini and *The Unfakeable Code*® by Tony J. Selimi.

end of an exhausting work shift or a quiet room with refreshment in some remote part of the hospital, which the busiest doctors and nurses never have time to utilize.

Another important issue to consider is how excessive control hinders flexibility in emergency response. Some healthcare organizations, usually in pursuit to control expenses, adopt dysfunctional approaches and principles.

If we look at living organisms, they display a hierarchical structure of systems, organs, tissues, cells linked by bidirectional communication and carrying out specific functions. The hierarchy delegates certain tasks to systems and organs at a lower level, while the central structures concentrate on an overarching control of the whole organism and other higher functions. When these structures, communication channels, and functions are disrupted, disease or death occur.

Similarly, an organization that adopts unidirectional communication (telling – not listening) and centralization of power, with time, becomes dysfunctional until it gets dissolved or absorbed by another organization.

For example, I have worked in hospitals where, to have approval of a shift beyond the contracted hours to be worked by bank/locum staff, it required filling a paper form and signatures by managers of two hierarchical levels before being discussed and approved at a weekly panel meeting, and a similar process was required to get that shift paid after it was worked; as you can imagine, the system generated innumerable delays in having these shifts authorized, thus leaving essential services often short staffed, and long delays and errors in paying staff, with increasing levels of discontent and a massive reduction in the pool of staff volunteering to work these shifts.

Failure to successfully delegate is known as micromanaging; as a doctor, being on the receiving end of this style of management can be another source of frustration. Paying more attention to this source of frustration can support the management of healthcare to develop even better programs by utilizing consulting and business coaching tools so that managers and doctors can work better together.

Another common planning issue is failure to consider the actual workload, the timing and deadlines of a myriad of nonclinical duties and adequately allocate time to carry out these tasks in doctors' job plans.

As a result, many doctors are having to deal with multiple overlapping deadlines, e.g., the need to complete tax calculations and present a tax return, the need to summarize the activities of the past year and complete an appraisal, the need to discuss a job plan for the coming year, plus deadlines around applications for bonuses, deadlines for presentations and courses, etc.

My ex-partner used to complain that I was *married to medicine* as he witnessed me dedicating so many hours of my "free" time to preparing for these work-related tasks ahead of overlapping deadlines.

While we can't change the national deadline for presenting a tax return, what we can do something about is to look at what prevents us from spreading other activities and deadlines throughout the year. After all, it would just be a matter of coordination and *bidirectional* communication; currently, departments establishing a deadline affecting a certain employee may have no visibility of what other departments do and no visibility of the individual's job plan, calendar, workload, and ongoing projects.

Moreover, some departments may occasionally communicate in the style of little dictators, imposing deadlines and mandatory actions upon others rather than asking for availability and arranging a mutually convenient and realistic timeframe.

Many of you would agree that receiving dozens of e-mails just telling you what to do and by when, with the expectation that you must just say yes, or otherwise, look bad in the eyes of your employer, maybe receiving further reminders of a missed deadline and having to justify why you didn't do it, like a little kid in school, is neither efficient nor effective.

The visionary in me believes that with full transparency and visibility of workloads and deadlines and with alignment of workloads to allocated time, the need for nagging e-mails and embarrassing conversations will be significantly reduced. Plus, this would also be a valuable tool for managers to always understand exactly how many doctors the organization needs.

In summary, there are some actions we can take to shift from continuous crisis management to successfully planning doctors' workload. Here are some suggestions:

- Have a consistent buffer of doctors.
- Have a wide-spectrum workload and workforce planning, which includes planning for predictable crisis and uncertainty.
- Adopt lean management styles and delegate more effectively.
- Have an efficient setup, sharing, and management of work calendars.

Before moving on to the next chapter, here is a message worth sharing:

Wide-spectrum workload and workforce management reduce stress.

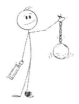

MATCHING COMPETENCE WITH DELEGATED AUTHORITY IS EMPOWERING

As doctors, we sometimes come across pop-up error messages on computer screens, such as "You do not have the authority to perform this task," "Access denied," "Access blocked by the administrator," "This task requires authorization by …," "Please get in touch with the system administrator," and the list goes on.

We all have encountered similar alerts in our personal lives; for example, when using computers other than our own, or even our own computer if we are not logged in as administrator, or when accidentally trying to access protected areas on a website. Am I wrong assuming none of you, my readers, is a professional hacker?

We may try to use different login details, change the security settings, or contact technical support; in some cases, we may give up and opt for an entirely different course of action.

But what if similar messages popped up when attempting to perform simple tasks in your job as doctors? Besides irritating you for slowing you down and making you less efficient, how would they impact patient care? Would it make them feel cared for? Would they feel like we respect and value their time? Would they have confidence in our professional skills and organization?

It is in answering these kinds of questions that we can start recognizing that there is a problem. In some healthcare organizations, this is a nearly daily occurrence; not necessarily in the form of pop-up messages on a computer, but in the form of having to waste time circumventing restrictions and rules that prevent some doctors from accessing certain diagnostic and therapeutic options for their patients.

The underlying reasons behind restrictions may vary from controlling expenses to controlling the use of resources that are considered scarce, controlling exposure to radiation and toxic substances, or controlling accidental confusion between items with a similar name, etc.

Often these control and safety systems are designed so that they impose more restrictions upon the more inexperienced members of staff and progressively less on more senior/trained staff members. If this design had ever been discussed in depth with the actual users, almost inevitably, they would have highlighted the following issue: Junior doctors are very often executing the instructions of a more senior and experienced doctor but find themselves without the system permissions to proceed with some of the simple tasks delegated by their senior, predictably resulting in avoidable delays.

For example, in a hospital I worked in, I regularly had to request certain blood tests neither the junior doctors nor the nurses were able to request following my plans. The question then becomes, is that good use of a medical consultant's time?

Even as a senior doctor with years of experience, I sometimes found myself unable to proceed with requesting a certain test or prescribing some medications, occasionally with no immediate solution because of this occurring outside office hours or because of the complicated layers of bureaucracy I was faced with to circumvent the restriction.

Some of the restrictions I encountered border on absurdity.[5] For example, in certain hospitals, some inexpensive and innocuous substances normally marketed as supplements that anyone can buy without prescriptions in health stores and supermarkets could only be prescribed by a limited number of specialists; while others, even if backed by scientific research,[6] had been removed from the formulary, the list of what is available for prescription in a certain institution/geographical area, as a way to reduce costs. The absurdity resides in the fact that while restrictions were imposed on something extremely cheap and completely safe, which is assumed to be futile, anyone with a medical license in the same organization was authorized to request certain very expensive tests or prescribe some very expensive drugs, including those that come with a long list of potential side effects and risks.[7]

I chose to share the above example not just as emblematic of the risible attempt to save a few pennies on a colossal healthcare budget, but also to bring awareness to another unseen negative consequence. At the time, I had just completed attending a series of international courses on nutrition and learned about the scientific research supporting the use of certain supplements and nutritional interventions. Yet I found my hands inexplicably tied in recommending the best course of action to my patients.

---

[5] The healthcare world is full of absurdities and paradoxes; it's not by chance that plenty of successful humoristic books and comedies drew inspiration from the medical world.

[6] Non-pharmaceutical research is often of comparatively smaller scale, lower impact, and frequently dismissed.

[7] I am aware that this opens a much wider ongoing debate around supplements, vitamins, guidelines, scientific research, etc., which is not the purpose of this book; therefore, forgive me for dropping the opportunity to expand and move on with other concepts!

When hitting these restrictions, what my internal critic[8] would hear was, "We, the hospital, don't trust you," "We don't think you are capable to make the right decisions for the patient," "We need to control the way you spend the money allocated," "If you want to use this tool, you need to ask someone *better* than you," "You are not good enough, we are taking this tool away from you," "Someone better than you has made this decision for you."

Years ago, no doctor would have shared this internal conversation, it would have been unthinkable, and if shared, it would only have attracted derogatory laughter. The good thing about today's medical profession is that we see more and more of us talking about and considering the emotional consequences of organizational actions on our well-being.

The positive aspect of a military-like style of communication in leadership is that there is clear accountability, and you know who issued the orders. However, many healthcare organizations adopt a corporate style of communication that conceals in anonymity the real decision-makers.

The language is almost always in the passive form and impersonal: "a decision was made," "the trust decided that …," "the board wants us to …," "the panel decided …," "the committee was advised that …"

As a result, nobody knows who the orders really come from and who to talk to in case of any serious issues arising. Often this kind of language is precisely what discourages doctors to give constructive feedback, leading to more frustrations and inefficiencies. Something I share more about in the following chapters.

Many doctors are not in favor of advocating for a completely unregulated and uncontrolled profession; in fact, it is the opposite. Doctors would benefit from regulations that are adaptable, flexible, and tailored to our ever-changing needs.

---

[8] If you are familiar with Eric Berne's Transactional Analysis, you will easily identify which part of my psyche heard this.

In honesty, majority of doctors mean well and want the best for their patients and the organizations they work for. Nevertheless, history teaches us that there have been, and there will be, a few that abused the power bestowed upon them and did harm. Unfortunately, the response to these events has often been excessive and at the same time ineffective, imposing a heavy burden of bureaucracy and restrictions on all doctors with numerous negative consequences and without really making it easier to identify and stop the few dangerous ones.

For example, it is often mentioned that Harold Shipman, also known as Dr. Death, would have probably passed with good outcome the revalidation process implemented as the very consequence of his nefarious actions. But at the same time, the cultural change that occurred in parallel would make it a lot more likely for coworkers to raise concerns at an earlier stage. And understandably, cultural changes are a lot more complex and ephemeral compared to policies and regulations.

Another paradox to tackle is the notion of having full accountability without full authority.

I have observed that doctors at all levels of experience and grade suffer the consequences of an imbalance between personal accountability and the degree of authority and self-determination they are allowed.

The level of accountability for doctors remains unparalleled and vastly unquestioned. For example, a doctor might have to respond to a complaint; might be reported to the professional regulator, who may start investigating their fitness to practice; might be reported to their line manager or other management; might be reported to the police; and might be prosecuted in a court of law for alleged civil or penal crimes. In a few unfortunate cases, all these can happen simultaneously.

Moreover, a senior doctor is expected to take full responsibility for the actions of all the doctors they supervise, regardless of whether they work with them steadily or only occasionally, which nowadays is the norm because of complex hospital-wide rotas and constantly changing teams.

While accountability and responsibility are full, the doctors will be rarely given full authority and independence, for example, to choose from all available investigations and treatments for their patients, to allocate the time they judge necessary to conduct a good consultation, to allocate adequate time to supervise and educate trainees and other professionals, to allocate adequate time to carry out administrative tasks for their patients and their departments, to influence budget allocations, to plan future developments of their departments, etc.

In other words, if doctors are not authorized to do all they can for patients, how can it be that they are asked to retain full accountability for what happens to patients?

Increasingly, doctors are vocalizing their demands. For example, that personal accountability needs to be accompanied and counterbalanced by organizational accountability, the external factors that prevent the individual from giving their best, to be fairly judged. Unfortunately, so far, organizational accountability often remains limited to finances, e.g., liability insurance, compensations, etc., and is not always taken into account in proceedings against doctors.

Another source of frustration worth mentioning is how in the same organization you may have members of staff with so much more power and independence and lower accountability than doctors. Something worth examining.

Here are some ideas worth considering for change to happen:

- Setting up authority and accountability levels to be proportional to competence.
- Simplifying access to diagnostics and therapies by removing obstacles affecting doctors' ability to investigate and treat patients.

Dr Pietro Emanuele Garbelli

- Involving doctors in the design of escalation processes to save time.
- Including doctors' feedback in crucial conversations that influence regulations.

Before you move on to the next chapter, here is another message worth sharing:

Every tradesman decides what to have in their toolbox. Why not doctors?

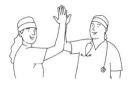

PUT YOUR CONFLICTS ASIDE: PATIENTS COME FIRST

In this chapter, my aim is to address another source of frustration that comes from playing power games that are no different from the ones we were subjected to when we were children.

"I'm going to tell the teacher what you did!" "You dropped it, you pick it up!" "They gave it to me first!" "My mom said I shouldn't play with you!" "I don't want it anymore!" "I didn't break it, it was him!" "Stop nagging me!" "But I don't want to!" "That's not my problem!" "My daddy is stronger than yours. He'll show you!"

Who would have expected kindergarten and primary school-style interactions to follow us well into adulthood and in the workplace?

Let's be honest: While nearly all interactions among doctors go smoothly, every now and then, a silly dispute arises and, if you listen attentively as an external observer, hidden underneath adult language, you can sometimes hear two kids fighting. Because of the hierarchical organization, and the usual recommendation to "escalate" any problem to your superior when you can't settle it yourself, we occasionally overhear or report conversations that sound like "I am going to tell my daddy/mommy (boss) that you refused to do X, so he/she will speak to your mommy/daddy (boss)," "I will need to speak to your mommy/daddy (boss) as you're being such a brat (unreasonable, obstructive, uncooperative)," "If you don't apologize, I'm going to tell Daddy/Mommy (report your behavior)."

Obviously, as an external observer/listener, it's much easier to read between the lines and notice the childish behavior in certain arguments among doctors; while when we are directly involved, our emotions may temporarily take over rationality, and we might engage in similar responses.

When under pressure and exhausted, many of us doctors, who may be perceived as calm, occasionally lose our temper; but what is our typical reaction when that happens? While we may intuitively acknowledge that nobody is expected to be a "saint," typically, we escalate (tell mommy/daddy) the lack of professional behavior and remind our colleagues about the standards of behavior expected by the regulators or the organization. But at what point do we press pause and reflect, asking ourselves the reasons why this behavior occurred and in what other efficient ways we can respond?

Because of the nature of our jobs, we rarely have the time to address the root cause of what we judge in others. Most of us doctors don't wake up in the morning thinking, "Today I'm going to be a total ****!" Deep down, we want to do our best. Keeping this in mind means it's important to address the underlying reasons why, rather than responding by blaming the individual(s) for what happened. In doing so, we can come to an understanding of the underlying causes and contributing factors, and by listening to what transpires, we can then ask *how* we can fix these "childlike" responses that waste time and create unnecessary frustrations for doctors.

For example, many factors can contribute to us choosing undesired responses or unconsciously negatively reacting to external stimuli: being tired, hungry, stressed, overworked, rushed, overstimulated, noise, aggression and other emotional triggers, not being listened to. Something as simple as identifying a few typical triggers that are more likely to make us "snap" at someone in our personal and/or professional lives can shine a light in the reasons why we respond the way we do.

We can surely reflect on what these triggers teach us about ourselves in an introspective journey. I highly recommend to do this with some external guidance initially.[9] But we can also influence the environmental factors that make us lower our tolerance threshold, such as reducing the noise level, minimizing interruptions, distributing the workload in a way that allows doctors to take regular breaks, etc. Nurses who typically work longer shifts are way ahead of doctors in this.

Another useful step is reflecting on why we are having an argument in the first instance; for example, is it because there are no clear rules about whose competence is to carry out a certain task or which specialty a patient with a certain pathology should be admitted under? "Fixing" such blurred lines may not be of your competence as a doctor and won't certainly be an instant solution. But it's definitely worth taking the necessary steps so that similar disputes won't repeatedly take place in the future.

If you are a doctor who has worked in hospitals long enough, you may have witnessed or been directly involved in some interaction that appears a "power game" among people belonging to different groups, specialties or professions. The question you may want to answer is, how do you react when someone refuses to do something for a patient and you perceive they are just being difficult?

Ideally, considering the possibility that your perception might be misleading could give you a head start. Have you succeeded in communicating exactly why you are asking for their help? Have you chosen the right person/specialty? Have you explained clearly what you need from them, which you may be unable to provide yourself to the patient? Do you have a broader understanding of their point of view?

---

[9] You can find further insight on what external triggers teach us about the parts of us we reject in *The Unfakeable Code®* by Tony J. Selimi.

I know we don't have the expertise or the time to dissect our own, let alone somebody else's, psychology. So the question I have for us all is, how can we resolve conflicts in a creative way? Many of us have experienced when fellow doctors go down a guilt trip ("Are you saying you are refusing to help me/the patient?" "Would you do the same if this were your mother/father?") and also observed others fully embrace playing the power game ("Can I please have your name and the name of your boss?" "I am going to document in the patient's notes that you are refusing to …").

What about using alternative ways to overcome conflicting situations? One of the tools I have successfully used to defuse conflict is humor; for example, after the request for a scan for one of my patients was rejected multiple times by the on-duty radiologist on a very busy morning, after two junior members of my team had discussed the details with them over the phone in two separate occasions, I went to the radiology reporting room of the hospital, and while opening the door, I announced in an exasperated tone, "Who do I need to *sleep with* to have this scan approved for my patient today?"

As I expected, among some faces who clearly expressed embarrassment (I practice in England, need I say more?), some of the senior consultants laughed and just politely asked me, "How can I help you?"

To be clear, I'm not recommending that you now all start going around your hospitals "bribing" every uncooperative colleague with sex jokes: I'm visualizing many noses starting to turn upward at this point. But just consider using humor mindfully and appropriately as a tool to defuse a tense situation and help restart a dialogue in a more productive way. In other words, make them laugh, and try again.

Another possible tool for us doctors to consider is explicitly admit that we are struggling and ask for help. Many of us don't show our vulnerability from the fear of undesired consequences. If you are like me, you may have learned to associate it with weakness, defeat, loss of control, cowardice, stupidity, ignorance, incompetence, and so on. But if we put our fears aside for a moment, we would genuinely ask for help.

For instance, asking along these lines: "I am really lost here, I don't know what to do for my patient at this stage, would appreciate your help." And we all feel great helping others. It is also an amazing opportunity for collaboration, mutual support, and learning.

And as usual, try to communicate in ways that others feel appreciated, listened to, and respected. Think about why what you are asking for would be important to them. How what you are asking for will assist them in their jobs or a situation that they may be presented with. What interest/benefit would they have? Try to put yourself "in their shoes" and observe the situation from their point of view. What is their concern? What in specific are they struggling with? What is it that you can offer to help them with or make their task less arduous? Can you meet them halfway? Most people will appreciate you asking curious questions that help them open up and safely be vulnerable.

While these tools are great, sometimes they may not get you the desired results. Occasionally, someone on the receiving end of the conversation might not be open to resolving conflicts without resorting to using power games, such as threats and punishments. Thankfully, if you as a doctor find yourself in situations like this, you can activate the existing official escalation channels.

Here is another thought to consider: Cultivating likeability helps you thrive as a doctor.

To be easy to relate to doesn't mean being a people pleaser, ignoring your needs, always saying yes, and trying to keep everyone happy all the time. What it means is to engage with people on multiple levels without adopting a rigid, monochromatic attitude in an attempt to appear "professional."

From personal experience, people tend to warm up and be open much more easily when we are relatable, and it takes considerably less effort than constantly trying to keep up the appearances and hide some traits of our authentic personality. For example, I noticed how other doctors started to open up and relate more with me and fellow colleagues when I was also being open about my experiences, challenges encountered, and mistakes I did as a migrant doctor at the beginning of my career. It helped us understand one another more and build better relationships a lot more easily than we would normally do.

Finding ways of relating to one another is also valid in building relationships with patients. For example, occasionally being open about shared experiences, such as having gone through the same test or procedure ourselves or having received the same diagnosis in the past, completely changes the way patients see us; as we find common ground as human beings, empathizing with their concerns and emotions and reassuring them, we end up building a two-way trust, thus enabling us to reach better outcomes for patients.

Assuming that disputes and tantrums are the exception and not the rule, some of you may be asking yourselves why bother investing time and energies in tackling these rare occurrences. The truth is it creates many long-term benefits.

First and foremost, we can prevent negative consequences affecting patients directly or indirectly, such as delays in admissions, getting specialist opinions, performing tests, establishing the correct diagnosis, and patients losing trust in the team/institution, which then leads to refusal of treatment, self-discharge or request of transfer to another organization or team.

Second, the well-being of doctors is improved. If we remain in a cycle of repeated conflicts, our stress levels go up, we resort to avoiding interactions altogether, we become more anxious, we display anticipatory defensive behavior, we become more aggressive and prejudiced, and we end up changing teams/hospitals constantly and hating our jobs and profession.

Who wouldn't want to work in a harmonious environment? We all strive to find the elusive ideal workplace: where we can thrive; where, when we incur difficulties, our first instinctual reaction is no longer one of blame; and where the environment, the organizational culture, is shaped by the role we doctors play and our potential to influence positively our colleagues/workplace.

Over the years, I have experienced many benefits working with Tony, a skilled life and business coach specializing in human behavior, who helped me realize how transforming deeply ingrained habits in ourselves as well as in the organizations we end up working for isn't a one-minute job. It takes time, commitment, and guidance.

It is why I recommend healthcare institutions utilize coaching, mentoring, and training as empowering tools to support doctors and their teams in their journey to excellence. A well-developed harmonious team can have positive rippling effects throughout the organization.

Before you continue to the next chapter, here is an idea worth spreading:

Use humor, vulnerability, and relatability to dissolve conflict and build harmony.

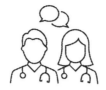

FEELING IGNORED? LEARN TO HEAR AND TO BE HEARD

A COMPLAINT I HEAR FREQUENTLY FROM DOCTORS OF ALL GRADES is the frustration arising from not being heard: "Nobody listens." "What's the point of filling another survey when nothing ever changes?" "What was the point of that long meeting when they haven't changed anything about the plan?" "We scheduled a one-to-one meeting, and they spent all the time talking about themselves and what they want me to do." "I've told the clinical director and the medical director too, but nothing has changed."

Sounds familiar?

As doctors, perceived as high-achieving individuals, at times we may find it challenging to get used to working in a highly regulated and hierarchical environment that offers a limited range of freedom. We have tremendous aspirations about what we can do and a desire to be consulted and involved in matters that affect us and our ability to provide high-quality patient care, yet when we perceive our opinions are disregarded, we end up frustrated.

We spend considerable amount of time to build our expertise and experience as doctors. We see the effects of the various decisions made by the organization we work in; thus, we are a great source to offer valuable advice to shape those decisions that affect us, the organization, and ultimately, the patients. Nevertheless, if you speak to many doctors, you will often be told how their voices are not being heard.

I found myself in similar situations many times. For example, in one of the hospitals I worked in, I was given the responsibility to set up a new department, which I did, but then without being consulted, a decision was made to move it to a different location shared with another service. As a result, patient care was disrupted, the productivity of the department dropped, stress levels increased, a lot of time was wasted in trying to address the additional problems created, and a lot of time was also spent to find suboptimal solutions to mitigate avoidable new risks. Furthermore, the morale of the whole team dropped, and the reputation as a healthcare provider and employer was damaged.

One decision made without doctors' involvement is all it takes to trigger bitter frustrations and negative emotions directed toward our superiors, colleagues and employers, which then contributes to creating dysfunctional work relationships, a climate of mistrust and antagonism, coveted rebellion or open confrontation and class action, frequent job turnover, and ultimately, doctors drop out, burnout, etc.

Now imagine the effect that thousands of such decisions being made without consulting us doctors would have on the effectiveness of the organizations we work for and the patients we are there to provide care for.

The truth is, even when we are being consulted, many times we find ourselves not being heard. So what can we doctors do to find ways to have a voice that is being heard?

The general assumption is that we are good communicators, but then why do many of us struggle to be listened to?

As doctors, we are trained to be good listeners. Why? Because our job is based on gathering information to make hypotheses (diagnoses) through listening and questioning. The degree to what good listeners we are varies a lot, depending on many factors,

Dr Pietro Emanuele Garbelli

among which personal experiences as a patient or paying attention to patients' feedback. But to what extent can we empower doctors to become excellent communicators when it comes to speaking?

Commonly, we concentrate on being able to explain medical issues clearly, avoiding medical jargon, adapting the language used, and checking that the patient has understood. Those of you with an academic career might have worked on improving your presentation skills, and most doctors will have worked on developing the skills to be great educators/teachers. But when it comes to public speaking or pitching an idea, many of us are generally out of our depths. This is important because when we participate in strategic meetings, we must be able to successfully present and pitch ideas. And when asked about our opinion or initiating conversations, we need to be able to capture the listener's attention and influence decision-makers.

If you are like me, most likely nobody taught you those crucial skills that we as doctors need to have to hear and be heard. We all have heard fellow doctors or healthcare professionals who don't do it well in conferences and meetings we attend, so why is it that we expect them to be heard? Improvising ourselves as speakers and influencers without investing in developing these skills is precisely what turns us into clumsy speakers like we judge others to be. And funny enough, that was the feedback I received from my coach Tony when he first asked me to record testimonials on camera or make an announcement and practice for a public speech. The truth is I perceived it as *the most painful thing* I had to do in my life! In each session, he would help address all the fears, doubts, and train me on how to structure, present, and clearly communicate my ideas so others would be inspired. Frankly, it is like going to the dentist and expecting to have a tooth extraction without anesthesia, imagine that?

What changed?

I learned to express myself authentically, organize my ideas, pay attention to pros and cons, and be able to handle objections better. Instead of going to a meeting with preconceived fears, feeling disempowered and anxious, I now look forward to going to meetings feeling calm, empowered, and heard.

Looking back, I never expected myself to be able to do this so naturally. Has it been a gradual change? Yes. Did I have to do a lot of work? Yes, I did. Paying attention to what I think and what comes out of my mouth has been of priceless value to me and something I believe all of us doctors would benefit from. So let me share a couple of things I have learned.

When others talk, learn to listen attentively.

What that means is we can train our brain to stop formulating answers or questions while someone else is speaking. And when we do this, not only the person who is talking to us feels heard, but also, they are more likely to do the same for you.

As doctors, we often assume just because we work together in healthcare, we share the same interests, beliefs, and values; for example, taking care of our own and other people's health, their safety, and what equipment we may need to do our jobs well. We assume everyone should automatically agree with our point of view and expectations of what is best for our patients, and we get angry when they don't agree. We get incredibly frustrated and start blaming others as they "don't listen," "don't get it," or "don't care." Sounds familiar?

I found myself in the same situation many times and vented my anger in my private coaching sessions, where instead of the reaction we are used to hearing from our friends ("Oh those ******, poor little you!"), I was invited to look within, reflect, listen to feedback, and learn.

The assumption that we all share the same ideas couldn't be farther from truth: Each of us as unique individuals has a different set of beliefs, priorities, and ways we look at and interact with the world. When interacting with others, it is therefore important to express our opinions in a way that makes sense for them and captures their attention; in practice, this means putting ourselves "in their shoes," i.e., we are listening to ourselves from *their* point of view. You'll be surprised how much you learn about what really makes people tick.

If you want to be heard, understand who you are speaking to.

To put it simply, we need to adjust the content of what we are trying to communicate according to what is important to the listener.

Sometimes we speak to a group of people assuming they have things in common, but in fact, they don't. For example, other doctors will be more likely to be on board with you regarding a certain proposal when you engage them in ways that support them; e.g., improving patient care by reaching accurate diagnoses more rapidly, reducing medical errors, simplifying the administrative passages. On the other hand, nurses in your department may be more interested to hear how what you are saying is going to benefit them; e.g., more time available to spend with patients providing care, less complaints by carers, receiving clearer plans. Managers might be interested to hear from you yet another set of benefits, such as reduction in medical errors, length of stay, complaints, legal and settlement costs. Remember to, first and foremost, understand who you are speaking to.

If you have ever written a business plan for a hospital you may be working for, you will have noticed that you are guided to implement a similar process listing all the implications of the proposal, the benefits and drawbacks, the costs and savings associated, and how it would impact a range of other departments, services, and professions.

Applying the same principles in verbal communication is a skill that doctors can hugely benefit from.

Stop telling, start asking.

Another mistake we commonly make when communicating, in particular when being antagonized or questioned about our ideas/ proposals, is that we engage our "dictator" persona and start teaching and *telling* people what they *should* agree with, do, or know.

If we are honest with ourselves, deep down, we *hate* it when someone tells us what we should do or what we should agree with. However, occasionally, we all find ourselves unconsciously doing the very same thing to others, only to get angry when they stop listening.

A nonconfrontational way to lead someone to agree with something that is of benefit to both of us is asking open-ended questions; it is said that asking powerful questions is the quality of a master.

When asking questions, one attitude to definitely avoid is assuming that we know what they need. So what kind of questions could we ask instead? Ideally, asking questions helps the listener realize how something we are trying to communicate is of benefit to them. You can use metaphors, examples, or questions, such as "Have you thought about this?"

Observing Tony skillfully using this technique to defuse challenges and antagonism is a very interesting and humbling experience, and my initial reaction was, "I'll never be able to do that!"

But as I am learning to be better at it, I realized more its transformational power.

How to apply this principle of stop telling and start asking is a mastery on its own. It is a wonderful practice that offers us doctors endless possibilities.

Turn personal attacks into purposeful change.

We occasionally encounter certain people who might be absolutely determined to antagonize us at all costs, even attack us publicly. Although there is a framework around handling physical attacks, what we are not prepared for is how to respond to public intense criticism that damages our mental well-being.

One possibility I hadn't considered, which was suggested to me by my coach Tony when reflecting on how differently I could have responded to a personal attack, is to just say "You are right."

Think for a moment about how powerful this simple statement is. Although our egos may find it very challenging to say them, these simple words can placate someone instantly. When someone is engaging in their animalistic fighting behavior, one possible response is to drop to their level of communication and attack back, or we can choose to placate the animal in them by throwing them a steak, metaphorically, and move on.

In other words, we can tame our pride and desire to want to be *right* all the time for creating a moment of peace and the ability to move on swiftly to another conversation.

Stop speaking of what you don't want and focus on what you want.

If you pay attention, one of the most common behaviors people show when asked "What do you want?" is to start listing everything they can think of that they don't want.

This is something I too was unaware of; whenever my coach Tony asked what I wanted, I unconsciously used to start listing what I did not want. He kept insisting for me to tell him what I want, and I kept telling him what I don't want. The truth is I honestly had no idea I was doing it and where I learned this behavior. But since

Tony kept repeatedly pointing out to me each time I was doing it, eventually, I really started to pay attention to it. I made it my focus to do it a lot less and catch my own thoughts before even speaking them.

You may wonder, why does this matter? Because, to put it simply, you never get what you want by speaking of what you don't want. Moreover, I used to immediately lose the attention of the person I was talking to without understanding why.

This principle applies also to when we moan in our workplace.

So before we move on to the next chapter, let me leave you with the following question:

Why not focus our conversations on the things
we want that can make a difference?

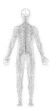

THE ART OF MEANINGFUL FEEDBACK

ONE REMARKABLE COMMON DESIGN IN LIVING BEINGS IS THE existence of feedback mechanisms, whereby information flows in two opposite directions; for example, the brain sends commands to various organs, while sensors in those same and nearby organs inform back the brain, not only about the actual execution of the command, but also of a multitude of other information.

Our brains receive a plethora of input from sensors located within the body and at the interface between the body and the external environment (the "five senses" we are used to recognize), automatically, unconsciously, processing most of that information by filtering, sorting, reacting to it, adjusting command signals; and only a fraction of all that information reaches our consciousness every now and then.

Other well-recognized examples of feedback mechanisms allow the maintenance of relatively constant characteristics within the body in terms of chemical composition, temperature, pH, dissolved gas levels, hormone levels, etc. Information is constantly exchanged and acted upon to simply maintain our bodies alive and in perfect working order.

It isn't, therefore, a surprise that many machines and systems designed by engineers embed similar principles, adopting feedback loops and bidirectional communication channels.

With our knowledge and expertise as doctors in analyzing the functioning or disruption of feedback mechanisms in the body as a way to diagnose disease and identify ways to restore health, why is then our input in designing, assessing, and improving systems, technology, and healthcare organizations seldom taken into account?

What common "diseases" can we doctors identify in the organizations we work in, which decision-makers can use as essential information for improvement and efficiency?

A repeated pattern I observed in many organizations I have worked in is an issue with the "neurological" system of the organization leading to inefficient flow of information. Just like the body requires information to flow both ways, from the center of control, the brain, to the peripheral organs and vice versa, imagine how a similar architecture allowing efficient bidirectional information flow would greatly benefit organizations.

A common perception many of us have is that the information flows efficiently from the top down through the hierarchical structure, while it rarely goes the opposite way. In reality, the distribution of information from the top down is also often suboptimal; for example, we seem to invariably struggle to send out e-mails to all intended recipients.

Healthcare organizations are very dynamic and inevitably permanent, locum, and agency staff members join and leave throughout the year, and our support systems are not designed to efficiently keep up with this and keep an accurate and up-to-date record of staff members in all the systems the organization uses. In most hospitals I have worked in, doctors who had retired or left months or years earlier were still appearing in drop-down menus of electronic records, in distribution lists, and a myriad of other programs and systems, while new members of staff were nowhere to be found for weeks or months after joining, often requiring us to select a different doctor's name just to be able to carry out a certain task. This has obvious negative repercussions down the line; for example, after that particular task has generated a result that is communicated/attributed to the wrong doctor.

A common solution organizations implement to address the issue of information distribution is to publish vital updates and documents in their intranet; unfortunately, if as users we don't know there is a need to search for new information (i.e., we have not heard/been told that there has been a change), we won't think about finding that piece of information. And we cannot just rely on people randomly noticing things on a webpage by chance.

Another common solution implemented is sending bulletins to *all* members of staff as normally, global distribution lists are more reliable than those based on profession and departments. A problem with this approach is that people easily feel overwhelmed by the plethora of information they are bombarded with, and the risk is they might miss the few bits relevant to them.

But let's also look at the other side of the problem: bottom-up information flow, a very common source of frustration for us doctors.

Why does this matter? Doctors are in continuous direct contact with patients and other healthcare professionals; unlike the sensory organs of the body, we are the part of the organization that can not only sense what is going on, but also analyze the information, identify a problem and the need to inform the decision-makers about this. Unfortunately, we then often struggle to find ways to adequately communicate these problems because of the absence or inefficiency of bottom-up communication routes. Besides the frustration arising from the difficulties we encounter in identifying ways to pass on vital information, we also worry about the consequences of lengthy delays in addressing the issues we have identified and how that continues to impact patients and the organization.

Areas in which I have observed this working well in organizations I worked for is risk management and incident reporting. For instance, when it comes to recording, communicating, processing, and acting upon vital information regarding threats and incidents that have already occurred, we usually have efficient ways to handle this information using dedicated risk-management software and teams.

When it comes to other forms of feedback or information that the organization would greatly benefit from (doctors' feedback), we are usually not well prepared. Our institutions usually rely on doctors taking the initiative to talk to one another and their line managers or on infrequent surveys, which usually adopt a rigid structure composed of closed questions and little or no opportunity to add further information.

The subjective experience of us doctors facing these surveys varies; some welcome the opportunity to finally be given the chance to say what they think, hoping their answers will be listened to and make a difference in improving what is currently not working well. Nevertheless, in my experience, doctors who have compiled several surveys over the years end up disheartened when they haven't received an acknowledgment of the issues reported or seen any attempts to fix them. While there have been some improvement in incorporating staff engagement surveys, the truth is the response rates struggle to change from year to year.

Without efficient and reliable ways to report problems from the bottom up, the frustrations among doctors experiencing daily problems will usually continue to mount until some of the more vocal doctors find ways to be heard, usually venting out their frustrations in an outburst at the first practical occasion; for example, a meeting organized to discuss something else. Sounds familiar?

One cannot help but wonder if it is in the interest of the organization to leave doctors to accumulate frustrations like a pressure pot, or would it rather be more valuable to collect information as soon as a problem leading to frustrations is identified?

Doctors are so used to "swallowing" frustrations that if we are asked out of the blue, out of context, to tell which problems we encounter in our jobs, initially, we would only be able to mention a few. But in reality, we have hundreds of problems that at that moment we simply forget about. Given the opportunity to talk for a longer time, many more problems would come to our mind. If we were invited to think about all the problems we encounter over an entire day at work, we most likely would be able to identify many more.

But what positive changes would happen if we could make a note of problems and frustrations at the very moment they arise?

Most of us are used to make mental, physical, or electronic notes of important thoughts to ensure we act upon them at a later stage. Our smartphones, computers, and other electronic devices include functions to support us with these tasks. Some of us already make notes of issues we want to communicate later on in an e-mail. But what about designing a much more comprehensive solution? For instance, we could implement some sort of instant feedback capturing mechanism that would allow us to identify *all* problems occurring in the workplace in real time. Imagine that?

A few years ago, capturing, processing, and interpreting real-time information would have been impossible. It would have meant employing a lot of people just to receive, record, read, divide by category/department/urgency, etc., and then manually direct information throughout the organization.

It is why companies employ more and more advanced technologies to shift tasks from humans to machines; we *reluctantly* got used to speak/chat to machines when contacting most customer support lines, we scan our own groceries' barcodes, check-in our luggage at the airport, etc. What we often don't realize as customers is what goes on "behind the scenes" involving recording, processing, storing and using information, eventually making certain functions automatic and making our lives a little bit easier. For example, our favorite supermarket "knows" our preferences and what we usually buy, so we might find those products more easily when shopping online, and we may receive suggestions for similar products when the one we usually buy is not available.

Similarly, information handling in our work environment as doctors can be automatized and applications for electronic devices can be made available to doctors to capture data. This can then become a very useful tool in designing optimal systems that doctors and everyone involved in providing healthcare can use.

Ideally, an optimally designed system is one as unobtrusive and lean as possible, requiring as little user effort as possible. Artificial intelligence is becoming a major player in data capturing, handling, processing, self-correcting, identifying patterns, and proposing solutions. It has the ability to use the data captured with existing technology (cameras, microphones, keyboards, etc.), but paired with even more sophisticated interfaces, it would reach a much higher potential.

For example, with current technology, we have the ability to give software companies real-time feedback about the functionalities of their software just by clicking on a button or letting them have information about what went wrong when their software crashes automatically. Similar functions could be included in our hospital software systems.

So what could future technology look like? Smartphone apps could be developed to allow us to report frustrations and problems. But why stop there? Imagine how useful would be to have a holographic or robotic assistant that listens, notices your problems and frustrations, and is able to automatically transfer that data upstream and generate solutions. For doctors, it would be priceless!

What information could we collect?

The possibilities regarding what information we could collect are endless; in my opinion, simply everything that frustrates doctors, employees, patients, regulators, and everyone involved in healthcare.

While current systems capture information partially and inquire about preconceived impact hypotheses, a comprehensive approach to feedback would reveal how in organizations, just like in living organisms, every part influences the whole. Healthcare organizations would be empowered to improve decision-making, being able to see the real impact of any change at every level of the organization. Especially, it would reveal the hidden impact of decisions that create unnecessary frustrations for us doctors and ultimately increased costs.

For example, we would be finally able to see the real impact of outsourcing services, not only on the quality of the service provided (cleaning, sterilization, catering, imaging, etc.), but also on doctors and everybody else's efficiency, productivity, and well-being.

Hospitals tend to outsource more and more services to external companies, therefore reducing the number of employees and costs; but often what goes unnoticed is the drawbacks of this decision. As out-of-hours services are more expensive, whenever possible, outsourced services are usually contracted to work in office hours.

But why does this become an unnecessary frustration for us doctors?

Let me share with you what happens on a typical morning ward round nowadays. Doctors will attempt to see patients while they are being served breakfast and orders for their lunches and dinners are being collected. At the same time, the floors are being vacuumed and mopped, the fire alarms are being tested, the curtains are being changed, and sinks and toilets are being unblocked. And at times there might be some construction work taking place, inspections, visits, and audits carried out.

As you can imagine, even if doctors were not expected to maintain a high level of concentration and attention to detail, including being able to communicate effectively and being able to hear some feeble internal body sounds, they would quickly become irritated by constantly being surrounded by noise, disruptions, and distractions. Often fellow doctors would describe this as being expected to work in a "zoo-like" or a "street market" environment.

Is this chaos unavoidable? Probably not entirely, but for the most part, it is. I worked as a medical student and as a junior doctor already at times when many services started to be contracted out, but I remember I could follow ward rounds without continuous interruptions and distractions.

A chaotic environment does not only affect the doctors and other healthcare workers, but also, ultimately, the patients, who not only are indirectly affected by our inability to be at our best but also complain about high noise levels throughout the day and most importantly at night, frequent interruptions, being frequently moved from place to place, etc. We often collect patient feedback, but when do we stop and reflect on what they are trying to tell us, and what we can do to make their experience better?

When planning has already occurred and these issues come to our attention in the form of feedback, it's a great opportunity to revisit these decisions and, for example, renegotiate some details of a contract or schedule activities differently throughout the day to minimize overlapping and negative impacts.

What can we start doing more of?

Using the systems we already have in place to start sharing our feedback, familiarizing ourselves with the structure of our organization, the "who's who," the various departments, who is in charge of different aspects, and communicating the issues we experience/notice they might be unaware of. We already have e-mails, telephones, meetings, and you might already have access to other smarter tools you can utilize.

As healthcare providers, it is in our common interest to make the organization we work for successful. Our feedback can help implement smart information management systems. If that is your remit, consider suggesting this in your organization, sharing some examples mentioned in this book of how this would benefit them at multiple levels.

Implement Bidirectional Feedback

If you are at the receiving end, don't forget to "close the loop" and communicate the effect of the feedback to the very same doctors who reported the issue. As previously mentioned, doctors soon lose interest in engaging in feedback unless they see that their efforts have tangible consequences.

The organization you may be working for might already be sharing some examples of responses to the feedback received in their newsletter or departmental bulletin. We see examples of this in some newsletters using phrasing such as "You said … we did" or "We listened …"

Ideally, you may want to contribute to the implementation of a tighter loop, making sure the information reaches the same people who have generated the feedback in the first place so that there is a direct link. This increases trust between doctors and employers.

In some cases, we already have the tools to be able to close the feedback loop, but we might not be using them. For example, the risk-management software might already have a functionality that enables us to send a feedback message to the person who originally reported a problem. Unfortunately, because of the number of reports received and the scarcity of resources allocated to process them, what we often end up receiving is either no message or an automatic message informing us the case was closed. This generates frustration; in changing this, we can build trust and engagement.

Other useful functions of bidirectional feedback are to identify and reward talent in your organization; good ideas can come from anyone, regardless of the job they were employed for, and they most likely gladly and enthusiastically would join a project to develop that idea into reality.

Feedback can be passive (anyone can send it at any time) or active (for example, before implementing a change, or afterward, or in response to an event), generic or specific, relevant for just a small service or group or for the whole organization. It is, therefore, essential to invest some energy, time, and money into managing it correctly and making good use of it, exploiting all its potentiality.

We have become accustomed to receiving requests for feedback from most businesses following each purchase/service, and many surveys reach our inbox periodically, to the point that we develop *survey fatigue* and stop engaging. How do we avoid making the same mistake?

Concentrating on facilitating spontaneous and ad hoc feedback helps doctors and other people give feedback promptly so healthcare organizations can make decisions that make things right for everyone.

So let's look at the options to make spontaneous feedback easy.

Let's be honest: Many ways that have been designed so far to replace human input put an excessive burden on the user, from selecting among multiple options in long drop-down menus to navigating multiple layers of vocal menus in an automatic answering system. Who hasn't, at some point, cursed the programmer/company/machine in question and desperately tried to find ways to speak to another human being instead?

Nevertheless, some "behind the scenes" technology can occasionally surprise us. For example, when as a result of me shouting "I want to speak to a human being!" or something similar to a helpdesk voice-recognition software, I was actually connected to an operator, although it was none of the options listed. The AI algorithm must have recognized my request. Sooner or later, we will see implementations of AI in healthcare, so we may as well work together to design solutions for optimal feedback handling.

Another limitation of the systems currently in use is that they are totally dependent on (the illusion of being able to) preemptively making assumptions about all possible eventualities. Who hasn't found themselves unable to find an option that corresponds to their situation/need? Occasionally, those who designed the system also "forgot" to give "other" as a further option, forcing us to either give up or choose the wrong option.

Ideally, AI will make such design mistakes a memory of the past and eventually allow for a more user-friendly interface that will also have the skill to adapt to what was not preconceived.

Imagine how efficient and time saving being able to send our feedback just by using the vocal command "feedback" to the device we are using would be for us doctors. AI would then decipher the vocal message recorded, classify it correctly, and forward it to the right people in the organization.

In the meantime, well-trained humans outperform badly designed computer systems; although not easy to quantify, the true costs of bad performance of any informatic system replacing human input should be taken into account in the cost-analysis. Perceived monetary savings can be quickly offset by a drop in performance, reputation damage, mistakes, loss of know-how, etc.

It is not by chance that despite some first-line clunky technology implementation, all hospitals still employ very effective telephone operators dealing with internal and external communications; calling switchboard sounds something from a black-and-white movie until we work in or have to deal with a hospital.

Before we continue our journey to the next chapter, here is a message worth sharing:

Bidirectional feedback loops are an essential component to future-proof healthcare organizations.

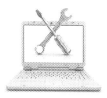

CAN'T WORK WITHOUT TECHNOLOGY? CARE FOR IT.

IMAGINE YOU LIVE IN A REMOTE PLACE WITHOUT ACCESS TO PUBLIC transport and rely on a car to take you to your job daily. When the car malfunctions, you have no choice but to promptly report the faults to a mechanic to have it fixed so you can continue getting to work. We see this as a natural behavior because it's our car and the only one.

Now imagine you work as a driver for a company that has a fleet of fifty cars. You are not the only driver, and you have no control over which car you are going to use at any time. Each time you pick up a car, you notice something not quite working the way it should, slowing you down in your tasks; would you be happy?

The company has a contract with a garage for the maintenance of these cars, and they expect you to report faults directly to them. You can't simply make an appointment and drop off the car at the garage, but you first need to report the problem online or via telephone. Each time you call, they keep you waiting for a long time, and the online form isn't quick to fill in either. When you are in a hurry, you end up switching cars and hope somebody else will deal with the faulty one. If all drivers did the same, what would happen to the fleet?

Very soon you would find one fault or more with nearly every car you pick, and it would become impossible to do your job. At this point, even starting to report all the faults becomes a challenge; all drivers complain about it, and everybody blames the mechanics for not addressing the problem. You always hear, "Our mechanics are terrible," but are they?

Like every profession, the practice of medicine has become more and more heavily dependent on computers (cars) that enable us to do our jobs. We might be still using paper here and there for records and forms, but the storage and exchange of the majority of information (scan images, laboratory results, etc.) have increasingly switched to digital, and most hospitals have or are in the process of adopting digital records, communications, orders, etc.

As the journey to digitalization is often progressive and not a once-off task, hospitals often end up utilizing a multitude of software products, more or less efficiently interfaced, requiring different specific details of software configurations on the workstations.

Some hospitals boldly invested in integrating as many functions under one single program/provider, thus resolving not only the obvious issues of compatibility and bidirectional information sharing (only partially addressed by the various ad hoc "integrations engines" that the IT departments deploy) but also the more obscure, but equally predictable, end-user problems with the optimal configuration of a single workstation, shared between multiple users, requiring very specific ever-changing configurations to run all the software in use.

Many other hospitals willingly or unwillingly take the route that is less visionary and daring in their IT investments and digital transformations. They maintain a plethora of systems in the impression this constitutes a money-saving, while often not realizing the real impact in terms of wasted time, reduced productivity, and patient safety.

As doctors, we need to access multiple results and documents to be able to make an accurate diagnosis, and our time is limited;

being slowed down multiple times per hour by constantly having to switch to a different PC because of IT glitches, such as being unable to launch a particular program or accessing a database is incredibly frustrating and unproductive. If you experience the same enough times in a day, you might soon be tempted to throw that computer out of a window. I often joke that's where the popular operating system takes its name from.

Most importantly, not having access to patient records and test results when we need them not only delays diagnoses and treatments but also exposes patients to preventable risks. Why rely on partial and potentially inaccurate information reported by patients and carers or on the interpretation of another doctor, when we could access the original data? Incorrect information could lead to administering a treatment that had already caused side effects/allergies in the past, repeating a test involving exposure to radiation/administration of contrast or other possible complications that could be avoided.

Hardware problems, such as a malfunctioning mouse, keyboard, printer, battery, etc., are equally frustrating and hard to solve. Sometimes the real issue might be not having clarity regarding who to contact and making sure the job receives the right level of priority. If not, a lot of users in a crucial area of the hospital can be negatively impacted.

Regarding software problems, identifying and reporting the issue correctly can be more challenging as they might show only depending on the program a user launches or on the configuration of a certain workstation or user profile. Ideally, once an identified issue is resolved, we would love to see the same solution applied to all computers in the organization rather than depending on independent problem reporting.

Fixing IT problems can't be a one person's one-off task, but it needs a collective iterative approach. For example, I have tried many times to arrange for an IT person to fix in one go all issues encountered on all PCs in a certain area of some hospitals I have worked in. Once it was all done, things seemed to work beautifully for a week or two, and then some problems started to arise again. I was shocked to notice how many things could go wrong in so many different ways in such a little time; after a few more weeks, the situation went back to square one.

The reason I am sharing this is to ponder on the following question: What other approaches can we have to improve the situation and positively impact productivity and safety?

At a national level, investing in unified digital health systems would have obvious benefits affecting all health organizations and users, being able to access past medical history, diagnoses, current medications, allergies and intolerances, test results, prescriptions, etc. It would greatly improve the efficiency of the health system at all levels, ultimately benefitting patients.

Sometimes I observe how astonished even elderly patients are when we let them know that we currently don't have immediate access to all their health information. All this while we all carry in our pockets devices capable to connect to information sources across the globe.

At a hospital level, this would translate into investing in unified solutions rather than patchwork interconnectivity for separate systems, adopting a reliable program to upgrade obsolete equipment timely, and deploying optimal configurations reliably, which benefits from standardizing the equipment and having a well-maintained directory of system configurations and unique requirements.

At an individual level, it's about collective shared computer maintenance responsibility. Our perception as doctors and nurses is often that we do not have time to report issues to IT, but at the same time, we forget that we end up wasting more time not doing so because more and more equipment becomes faulty. Learning to look after the equipment which we share and reporting faults promptly, our experience of using fit-for-purpose technology will drastically improve.

After all, we already make sure our personal stethoscopes are in working order, our pens are writing, our torches have charged batteries, and that we have all the necessary logins and passwords to be able to do our jobs, so let's go the extra step and, together, look after shared equipment better.

For instance, when I am in a rush, I snap a quick picture with my phone of the PC number and make a note of what doesn't work on that PC, then report it later when I have the time.

One thing that many of us doctors dream of seeing one day on the various software and hardware that we use is a "Fix Me" button. This would enable all of us to instantly report something not working without having to fill up forms, send e-mails, or phone a call center.

The Microsoft Word software I am using to write this book finally has a Feedback button, so why not every software we as doctors use?

Before you move on to the next chapter, here is a message worth sharing:

Being kind in the workplace is to show the machines a little love too.

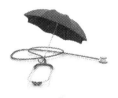

PROTECTING YOURSELF MATTERS: CHOOSE WISELY

My inspiration to write this chapter came from realizing the disparity that exists between patient's and doctor's protection.

The search for balance is innate within us, from the instinctual association of symmetry with "beauty" to the jealousy and rage against unequal treatment we surprisingly share with our fellow animals.

Following decades of medicine practiced in a paternalistic controlling way, and after a few exceptional cases of abuse of power and criminal conduct by few doctors, it is not surprising that the center of attention has been about protecting patients; numerous regulations and tools to ensure doctors' conduct is closely scrutinized were introduced.

With rare exceptions, I believe most doctors go to great lengths to protect patients, from providing health promotion and sickness prevention advice to screening programs for early diagnosis, to assessing the risk/benefit balance of each test, procedure, and treatment, to promptly reporting risks and incidents and implementing strategies to mitigate and minimize risks.

Where the patient's and doctor's protection pendulum of balance has swung too far is when we observe how healthcare employers, healthcare regulators, policymakers, patient advocacy groups, lawyers, and the police go further lengths and design systems to protect patients from bad doctors but do not protect doctors from abusive, aggressive and violent patients to the same extent.

For example, healthcare professionals report increasing rates of verbal abuse, threat and physical attacks from patients and relatives; this has sadly always been the case in some developing countries, but it raises concerns when occurring in highly developed countries previously known for the appreciation and respect the public had for their healthcare workers. For example, at the beginning of the COVID pandemic, healthcare workers were praised and clapped weekly, while at the same time or not much later, some of us were attacked.

A common practice for all hospitals is to have security 24/7, warning signs against abuse and aggression displayed in public areas, and panic alarms available in areas of concern to call for help promptly. We are also slowly seeing improvements in the care provided to us when victims of aggression, borrowing some expertise from institutions with more experience in the field, such as the military, police, etc.

One form of aggression doctors experience comes from being unprepared to deal with telephonic and online abuse. While we may be happy with the way security officers handle the occasional attacker, many of us find ourselves unprotected when the abuse comes via social media. What could be an easy solution?

Having been attacked on Twitter with many defamatory posts, I informed my back then-employer. What happened next made me feel unsafe. While they offered great protection against physical abuse, I realized there was no formal protection for verbal abuse, threats, reputation damage, and online abuse.

In cases like this, many of us feel forced to take matters into our own hands without much support from the very same institutions we dedicate our lives to work for. Furthermore, I was shocked to learn that Twitter did not consider the abuse I was subjected to as something that goes against their policies; thus, it was not something they would censor. Most of all, I was quite disappointed that the protection plan I had handsomely been paying for years offered just some basic advice, essentially admitting how powerless we currently are against these attacks.

Yes, I am aware that legal action can be taken for defamation, but wouldn't it be simpler and more logical to extend the protection provided by our employers and include these incidents in the protection policies we already purchase from medical protection firms and insurance companies?

Some forms of bullying and abuse come in the form of telephone calls, e-mails, and letters, so let me take this opportunity to say thank you to telephone operators, receptionists, secretaries, public relations, and communication departments for filtering the majority of these before they reach us doctors. Thank you for your service.

When it comes to patients, their relatives, and carers struggling to communicate with a certain department/doctor, they have, in some countries, the option to contact a Patient Advice and Liaison Service, i.e., a unique point of contact to resolve communication issues. Knowing how short-staffed certain departments are with unmanned telephones and unclear opening times, PALS offer an essential service bridging many gaps and allowing us to provide an answer to the most important concerns in a reasonable time. This service alone prevents escalation of the patient's, relative's, and carer's frustration into abuse and complaints.

Whoever works with the public knows how complaints are a two-edged sword: They provide important ways for patients and carers to raise concerns and for healthcare organizations to initiate investigations about incidents that might have gone unnoticed. They also provide another communication channel with the public which may reduce further escalation of disputes. Patients and carers have access to writing complaints and further requests for clarification to the response healthcare organizations send and the option to escalate the matter to an independent ombudsman if they are not satisfied with the response.

On the receiving end of complaints, healthcare organizations are required to abide by a framework that imposes rigid deadlines. Unfortunately, when doctors are required to respond to complaints, they might struggle to find time to do so in the timeframe required. Depending on the length, complexity, and volume of complaints, the time necessary to produce a response varies, and the support mechanisms provided by the organization may occasionally be minimal, requiring doctors to dedicate a considerable amount of time, diverting them from other activities. One way organizations could better support doctors and improve efficiency in complaints response is to employ adequate support—qualified complaints handlers. As a doctor, receiving a draft complaint response to work on frees our time that can be better spent on patient care.

Another major cause of doctors' frustrations comes from false allegations against us regarding our competence, safety, and clinical practice; anyone can report a doctor to their employer via several channels, to the regulator(s), to the police, and to civil or penal court of law. All these attacks, in some unfortunate cases, can happen at the same time, and doctors might suddenly face multiple parallel investigations on their practice. It is for this reason that doctors can purchase additional protection plans from mutual protection societies and insurance companies on top of the protection already offered by the employer.[10] Most doctors, concerned that the employer may be more concerned to protect themselves rather than the employee in certain cases, happily purchase individual protection plans, which also may include legal advice and coverage of legal costs.

Given the multiple types of possible attacks and scenarios, it would be wise to spend some time reading the small print and details of these contracts and policies and compare different offers, just

---

[10] This varies widely in each country; please refer to the regulations and medical protection offer in your country of practice.

Dr Pietro Emanuele Garbelli

like we do for our car insurance and other policies. In all honesty, we rarely do this until we find ourselves needing those services. Unfortunately, comparison websites, allowing us to quickly compare the essential aspects of these offers, do not exist for professional risks covers, making it much more time-consuming to find the ideal offer.

In general, mutual help societies may conveniently offer prospective and retrospective protection, i.e., not limited to the duration of the contract but prospectively offering assistance regarding incidents that occurred in the job/time covered by the contract, and may be competitively priced in comparison to similar protections offered by insurance companies. However, the cover may be discretional rather than full; this means that a panel will have the discretion to decide if they should offer help to defend your case or rather decline if they believe what you have done is undefendable, i.e., so different from what the majority of colleagues would have done in the same situation.

This opens serious concerns when it comes to the uncertainty of whether you would be covered each time you don't follow a certain guideline. As doctors, we know that guidelines are just general guidance based on some big studies about how to treat certain conditions, and we recognize the many limitations these documents and the studies they are based on have; for example, the fact that most studies do not include "real life" patients, such as those with multiple pathologies, the elderly, or those receiving multiple treatments for different conditions simultaneously. We, therefore, use the results of the study and the resulting guidance "with a pinch of salt," in conjunction with our baseline medical knowledge and clinical experience.

Nevertheless, in case of legal disputes, doctors are being more and more challenged for "not following" certain guidelines, and it has become doctors' common practice documenting in medical records the reason for not doing so.

But what would become of medical practice if we had to follow these principles by the book as if we were practicing law, documenting every single deviation from every single guideline all the time just to be sure we will be safe from legal proceedings?

Well, if you add to the time we currently take to see a patient and document in the notes, the time that it would take to produce 100 percent legally sound documentation, I estimate our productivity would pretty much drop by half. This could mean half of the number of patient visits per day or employing twice as many doctors to do the same amount of work.

In Utopia, a dual-trained medical and legal secretary could follow each of us doctors producing perfect medical records. But let's get back to planet Earth—what is possible is to have flexibility around applying different criteria in evaluating doctors' professional behavior in professional tribunals and in courts of law.

Another negative consequence of not addressing the issue of doctors not feeling safe is the increasing practice of defensive medicine. For example, requesting lots of tests and specialist opinions to minimize the chance of missing a diagnosis and to share responsibility. But doing so, we increase the chance for patients to be exposed to complications and to identify incidental non clinically significant findings, which then require further tests and procedures.

A defensive approach to medicine might also mean administering treatments even when the clinician is unsure of the diagnosis, using generic protocols and routines for everyone rather than attempting to tailor the treatment to the individual needs. Overall, it means waste of resources, increased risk, and lower quality of care.

It's smart to also be aware of the conflict that can arise between two opposite tendencies: on one side, technological advances that will allow us to analyze in great detail the patient's genetic material, metabolism, and microbiome, leading to a more tailored intervention, a.k.a. precision medicine; on the other side, guidelines relying on big-scale pharmacological studies recommending a uniform treatment for all patients with a certain diagnosis/characteristics.

Doctors practicing within regulated frameworks following official recommendations by professional bodies end up having a much higher degree of protection than those adopting approaches such as functional medicine or integrative medicine when it comes to defending their practice. This is because the same expectations are applied outside the field they were developed for.

The above distortions equally affect mutual support societies' panels, professional tribunals, and courts of law, while traditional insurance companies might choose to apply a higher premium when they perceive the practitioner has a higher-risk profile.

What are the consequences of incomplete protection?

The degree of stress doctors are exposed to when involved in proceedings against them, regardless whether by the employers, the regulatory bodies, the police or the legal system, is unmeasurable and has been implied in many life-changing events, including bankruptcy, long career breaks, mental and physical illness, career changes, and suicides.

Knowing that you could one day be involved too, particularly in absence of guaranteed full protections, can also be a significant source of personal stress, similar to the proverbial sword of Damocles; reading about high-profile cases in the news, witnessing colleagues' involvement, and reading newsletters from professional bodies, regulators, and protection societies can all contribute to living with a sense of impending doom, which cannot be healthy.

Before you move on to the next chapter, here are a few things to consider as a doctor or as a healthcare provider:

- Choose wisely the best level of protection for your individual circumstances as a doctor.

- Explicitly state and document the reasons for your actions, the clinical reasoning behind choosing a particular test or treatment.[11]
- Facilitate communication with everyone: colleagues, patients, relatives, other healthcare providers; so often litigation arises from assumptions, prejudice, misinterpretation, and distortion of communication, which could be settled quickly in a much less confrontational and formal way.
- Have more open discussions with our employers, regulators, and insurers about duties toward us as doctors and raise concerns when they fail to deliver.
- Report abuses promptly to all formal channels: security, line manager, risk manager, legal department, police, etc.
- Support fellow colleagues going through a difficult time, including crowdfunding of high-profile legal battles.
- Be aware that attacks are not only physical and verbal abuse but can also present as online defamation, bullying, etc.
- Join professional unions and advocacy groups and share your learning and experiences.
- Treat (protect) doctors like you treat (protect) patients.

---

[11] This does not necessarily mean going all the way to including citations of research articles and guidelines in our letters, as I have seen some colleagues doing

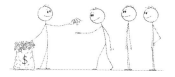

FEELING NOT BEING PAID ENOUGH? TOP UP.

"The sole purpose of money is to express gratitude."
—Tony J. Selimi

THIS CHAPTER WAS INSPIRED AS I REALIZED HOW DOCTORS AROUND the world, despite doing an incredible job, spending years to be trained, and saving lives, sometimes can't even get a mortgage to be able to have a home. I observed how many other professions that do not even require any formal training, education, or involve responsibilities for human lives are paid not double, triple, but in many cases, hundreds and thousands of times more than us doctors.

Furthermore, doctors' salaries vary widely in different countries; some of these differences depend on the exchange value of the local currency, some may depend on the nature of the workplace (e.g., public versus private healthcare), the reimbursement system, or the overall cost of healthcare in that particular country.[12] Doctors in certain countries will also incur higher expenses to cover for insurance and litigation costs.

Nevertheless, if we take into consideration the buying power of that salary, i.e., compare it to the cost of living and the average

---

[12] Which does not automatically correlate to the quality of healthcare, by the way, as measured on the basis of health indicators of the population.

salaries in that particular country, we still observe a wide variation. In other words, doctors are not being paid much in certain countries, but in other, countries they are.

This disparity certainly contributes to doctors migrating to other countries, although it obviously isn't the only factor. For the countries of origin, which often will have invested vast amounts of money on doctors' education, this equates to a continuous hemorrhage of workforce and talent.

Certain countries attempt to put in place restrictions to doctors' emigration or immigration accordingly, while others allow free movement or actively encourage immigration brought about by shortages in the profession by offering incentives. It still baffles me that in many countries, the number of doctors trained by the universities does not match the actual need that the country is predicted to have, with some countries training more doctors than they will be able to employ and others training less or significantly less, therefore continuing to depend on doctors trained elsewhere.

A question worth pondering is, what other benefits beyond our salaries do we doctors have that we don't see?

Depending on the healthcare system we may be working in, there might be further gains, discounts, bonuses, gifts, protection plans, reserved accesses, pension and healthcare contributions, tax deductions, etc., which all constitute forms of wealth we are usually "blind" to.

For example, in some countries, it is normal practice and even expected for patients to bring gifts or money to a doctor, while most Western countries regard this practice at high risk of inequalities as the wealthiest patients could gain advantages over others with bribing and, therefore, discourage or forbid this. From a point of view of a doctor with a small salary working in those countries, many would resort to welcoming the extra income.

Regarding bonuses, these are at first sight not as common in public healthcare as in the private sector or the corporate world, e.g., productivity bonuses, incentives, etc. However, many of us are unaware of similar bonuses existing in healthcare in other forms.

For instance, there may be small bonuses or prizes available for clinical, educational or research merits. Or it may be in form of schemes that support the purchase of means of transport (cars, bicycles, etc.) or technology (computers, phones, etc.), sacrificing part of the salary before taxes are applied. Further schemes might involve access to discounts locally or nationally; these are often not well advertised, and I regularly catch myself thinking I wish I had asked/checked when a colleague mentions they used a certain discount. The moral of the story is if we don't ask, we don't get.

Some of these discounts or schemes might be directly negotiated by our employers; others might be offered by organizations we are already members of or might be available at a national level for all doctors.[13]

Another example, during the COVID-19 pandemic lockdown, while we quickly grew tired of the applauses, we welcomed simple gestures, such as being allowed to skip a long waiting line outside a supermarket at the end of a grueling workday or free samples of food, drinks, and other products being distributed to us all in the workplace.

This is an example of how allowing more flexibility in the rules and regulations around receiving gifts and donations has a positive impact on doctors and healthcare workers, making us all feeling more valued at times when we put our lives at risk and contributing to keeping our productivity high and save lives.

We also feel appreciated and valued whenever people outside work treat us kindly. To this day, I still meet shop owners or other customer-facing employees who express their gratitude with extra kindness and attention when they find out about my profession; it might not bump up my salary but often makes my day.

---

[13] As these vary widely, please check with your employer(s) and professional organizations what is on offer.

Other hidden benefits are contributions our employers pay in pension schemes and national welfare (taxes), access to free education within the organization, contribution to expenses for external education. Compared to our self-employed colleagues, we have paid holidays and perceive a salary in case of sickness. With regard to sickness, the rules vary widely; and in some countries, it is possible to consider salary protection schemes to extend this benefit beyond standard contractual limits in case of prolonged or permanent sickness.

What we normally concentrate our attention on is the final salary, after deductions and taxes, and ways to increase it: career progression, increasing the hours we are contracted to work, working additional shifts within the organization, working additional shifts in other organizations (for example, via agencies), embarking in private practice (in addition, partially, or entirely). In general, all these options are only viable if we can endure the additional workload without incurring lots of stress and if we also cultivate likability and gratitude and, therefore, attract more business.

Most of us doctors receive no financial training, but at what cost?

Perhaps it is time for many of us to remove the blinders that stop us from seeing our salary as the only way to grow our wealth. One option is to make use of financial advisors specializing in advising doctors on saving strategies and investment opportunities.

For some of you, the phenomenon of doctor's entrepreneurship, which is getting increasing visibility, may be appealing. We used to be led to believe that only those of us making a *patentable* discovery in research would have had an opportunity to make money outside of medicine. The truth is, as I expanded my own awareness of what is possible, I realized how more and more doctors use start-ups in fields related to medicine (informatics, biotechnology, cosmetics, supplements, well-being, etc.) to complement their salaries. Others would use completely unrelated businesses, such as property development, entertainment, writing, etc., to grow their wealth.

After all, diversifying our sources of income benefits not only us but also our employers. For instance, being actively encouraged and practically supported in pursuing entrepreneurial journeys would reduce our constant search for better alternative employment and increase workforce retention. Furthermore, it would promote joint ventures, partnerships, patenting, trademark registration, and so on, benefitting the entire healthcare system. And that is an idea worth adopting.

You may want to start planning for regular savings and investments as part of solving the wealth-building piece of the puzzle. Why? Because when we perceive we struggle to provide for ourselves and our families, we live in a heightened state of stress which impacts all areas of our lives. Stressed employees have been shown to be less productive, make more errors, be sick more often, have a lower engagement, change jobs more frequently, and be less likely to show loyalty and dedication.

In other words, *well-paid, valued, and stress-free doctors are better doctors*, i.e., provide higher-quality care with reduced costs in the long term.

I trust all I have shared above stimulates your wealth-building creative juices. Here is a summary of things you can do as a doctor and as an employer:

- Look beyond your salary and recognize the multiple forms of wealth you have access to.
- Cultivate gratitude and likeability.
- Consider salary protection plans or equivalent.
- Get financial advice to invest and diversify your money.
- Pay doctors well, introduce reward schemes, and train them to look at the value received beyond their salary.

- Balance the costs of a higher salary against savings brought about by reduced sickness rates, turnover, locum/agency spent, litigation, insurance premiums, as well as increased productivity, retention, morale, and overall job satisfaction.
- Encourage and actively support doctor and healthcare organizations' entrepreneurship initiatives.

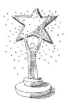

HONOR YOUR GREATNESS
AND THRIVE

"Be yourself, everyone else is taken."
—*Oscar Wilde*

AMONG THE MANY JOYS OF THE MEDICAL PROFESSION, HELPING younger colleagues overcome obstacles, grow, become better versions of themselves, and flourish in the profession is a beautiful thing to witness and a great reward.

The truth is we all play a role; whether we are aware, formally or informally, directly or indirectly, we educate and influence one another in a continuous cycle.

For this reason, we are often prompted and reminded to be *professional*, to be *role models*, to follow certain written or unwritten rules about what is expected of a doctor by the regulators and professional organizations and by our employers.

But have you ever felt there was something slightly off with this? Have you ever felt a resistance, an instinct, an inner rebellion, although you agree with those broad virtuous principles and expectations?

And similarly, have you ever felt you couldn't fully be yourself at work, being unable to say what you think or show certain personality traits? In my experience, these feelings are quite common in many professions and work environments, so why is it worth honoring our greatness and continuing to find more empowering ways to thrive?

Looking back at my studies and my career, I cherish many memories and stories about all the perceived good and bad teachers I had, and I am grateful to them all. Yes, the "bad" teachers too; let's humble ourselves and recognize that at times we all may be "bad" teachers but also that we learn by observing positive and negative role models. So why not use *all* opportunities presented to us to learn and become better teachers? Instead of focusing on teaching how *not* to do something, *not* to behave, *not* to think, or unknowingly challenge someone else, why not refocus ourselves to teach in ways that help us on our doctor's path by stimulating mutual learning?

Perceived "bad" teachers have helped us become who we are today as much as the "good" ones. Being supported and challenged each time we have been presented with obstacles has shaped our character, improved our critical abilities, and required skills to make informed decisions.

Without continuously overcoming obstacle after obstacle and learning from this process, we would all still be in our baby diapers. And without receiving help and nurturing, we would all be on a path that leads to premature death. Being supported and challenged are indispensable parts of continuous growth.

In the continuous process of learning and growth, we come across many influences. We might start the journey with some beliefs we unconsciously inherited from our family, culture, religion, friends, then absorb some from our teachers, professors, tutors, colleagues, employers. We encounter mentors, inspiring characters, figures of authority, antagonists, nemeses, negative examples and draw something from them too.

Like it or not, as we continue our evolution, our opinions, thoughts, and behaviors change. In some rare moments, we may notice how differently we used to think and behave once upon a time

Dr Pietro Emanuele Garbelli

and laugh at ourselves realizing how immature we now perceive our younger selves to be.

With all these external influences we are exposed to, we are left wondering, where does our journey to become more authentic start? And most importantly, what does it mean when we are told to be authentic? Is it even possible?

While there are great books to dive deep into these profound existential questions, for the purpose of this book, let's stick to the advantages of being authentic at work as doctors.

Let me start by briefly explaining why imposing our values on others does not work.

We all have been at the receiving end when someone insists we do something that we don't want to do. In *The Unfakeable Code®*, the author makes a brilliant case on how we can use a new style of communication to promote following rules and regulations. While being rewarded or punished may have worked in the past, a modern healthcare system would benefit from learning how to get doctors on board without *telling*.

When we get told, part of us feels restricted, uncomfortable, inauthentic, and squeezed in a box. At times the discomfort may be barely noticeable, like a constant grumbling underneath the surface, but at other times we may become aware of this discomfort when we "bite our tongues" and avoid saying loud and clear what we think. We, otherwise, may only become aware of the dissonance between our external behavior and our internal thoughts when we engage in introspection under the guidance of a counselor, therapist, or coach.

The less authentic we are, the less likely we'll also be to think freely, use our imagination and creativity, and communicate with others without the need to protect ourselves and hide our vulnerabilities. Instinctively, we tend to trust less people who we perceive to be inauthentic. As trust plays an essential role in establishing successful relationships with colleagues and patients, it is wise to avoid being stuck in this tricky situation.

We can be professional and authentic at the same time.

Yes, it sounds a bit confusing. Let me elaborate.

The paradox is that doctors are expected to change their personal behaviors according to a set of rules that in no way represents their professional expertise. This not only creates more frustrations, but it also encourages us to put on yet another "fake identity" that makes us feel caged, inauthentic, and eventually hate and leave the profession we love.

To alleviate this, let the uniqueness and even the quirkiness of your being show through the seams of that framework. You can learn not to worry about "what will people think," being judged, not being liked by everyone, sounding or looking different.

In all honesty, the most interesting and inspiring people I have met in my professional life, whom I still remember with a smile and longing, were not only very good healthcare professionals, mentors, educators but also uniquely singular and fascinating human beings not afraid to show all their wisdom and silliness, profoundness and laughter, politeness and rudeness; in short, showing both sides of the coin is what inspires others to shine bright.

We spend a lot of time worrying about what others think of us, but let's be honest: We can't please everyone. It is physically, statistically, and practically impossible to please everyone. No matter how much you try, there will always be someone who will judge you for what you stand for, be it your thoughts, your behavior, your appearance, your choice of clothing, the way you speak, your education, whatever.

Instead of investing energy in the unrealistic pursuit of pleasing and meeting other people's expectations, why not putting that energy into being your most empowered self and in what makes you thrive as a doctor?

And when what matters to you, your values, is in alignment with your workplace's values, imagine what synergistic explosion of creativity can happen.

Although workplaces often give the impression that we all are replaceable cogwheels, that the advertisement for our job will be published as quickly as we leave just to fill a generic gap, that nobody expects us to be anything special, in reality, every team and organization is thirsty for talent, for people with new ideas, for people who bring special qualities nobody else has and help everyone be more authentic. Why don't we honestly write this in job descriptions and adverts?

The special gifts you as a doctor may be able to bring to any healthcare organization are infinite. While we may not all make the discovery of the century that will revolutionize medicine, what you bring to your colleagues and your patients is unique to you, be it your wisdom, your personality, your many technical skills or "soft" skills, and the list goes on.

Next time you find yourself doubting if you have anything special to contribute, take a pen and paper, or open a Word document, and regardless of whether only you or others share those qualities and traits, start writing down everything you can think of that you do, that you can do, that you have done over the last day, week, month, year, decade. Keep writing, and then look at the pages filled with words. Do they awaken in you the feeling of gratitude? Do you *see* your magnificent self? If not, keep writing until you do.

For example, when preparing for my yearly appraisal or updating my curriculum vitae, I am forced to look back and list all the things that I have done in a year or longer. Often I start the process thinking I didn't do anything special, but the more I end up digging deeper through my records to retrieve what I have written, the e-mails I've sent and read, the notes of various projects, meetings, courses and conferences attended, etc., the more I start to observe how I've accumulated a list that goes way beyond what my initial observations were.

In doing so, this feeling of gratitude arises and makes me feel proud for all I have done. That's how you too can awaken your gratitude.

Remember: *Empowered doctors promote excellence and a collaborative spirit that plays a crucial role in Purposefully Transforming Healthcare*.

Thank you for coming on this journey with me.

Dr. Pietro Emanuele Garbelli

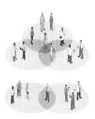

NEXT STEPS

I TRUST YOU GOT PLENTY OF VALUE FROM READING THIS BOOK AND it helped you identify how to make the most of your professional life as a doctor.

Here is what you can do next:

1. Invest in booking a Purposefully Transforming Healthcare® Consultation.
2. Book me to speak at your event to educate and inspire your audience.
3. Interview me and educate your TV, radio, podcast show, journal, or magazine audience.
4. Write a review on Amazon, etc. and help fellow doctors grow.
5. Sign up for my *Doctor's Empowerment* newsletter.
6. Connect and follow me on social media.

ABOUT THE AUTHOR

Trained in medicine across Italy and the United Kingdom, Dr. Pietro Emanuele Garbelli is a consultant physician specialized in acute internal medicine with an interest in medical leadership, bedside ultrasonography and integrative medicine. As a founder of Transforming Healthcare Ltd, he uses the wealth of knowledge and experience gained over many years to contribute toward shaping and purposefully transforming the future of healthcare.

After gaining his primary medical degree in Milan, Italy, he specialized in acute internal medicine in Florence, Italy, before moving to London, UK, where he broadened and honed his clinical skills. Over the following years, he continued to gain work experience in several hospital settings and in different medical specialties as part of a training program while gaining further local medical qualifications. After working as consultant acute physician and clinical lead for ambulatory emergency care, he successfully took on a role as clinical director for acute medicine.

Besides attending conferences, clinical and medical leadership courses tailored for the stage of his medical career, he embarked in parallel in an articulate journey of continuous self-development encompassing several disciplines, institutions, and teachers.

Growing up in a small town in Northern Italy in the late '70s, as a boy struggling to fit in an environment full of prejudices, Pietro's journey wasn't an easy one. While his close family provided a nurturing safe environment and plenty of intellectual stimulation, as soon as he started mixing with other kids at kindergarten and in the neighborhood, he was faced with bullying and homophobic abuse.

He did not understand why some kids called him names such as "sissy," "faggot," "pouf," "bent," etc.; at this stage in his life, he did not know the meaning of those words and did not understand why they were used as emotional weapons against him. His mother, Mariagrazia, was the only person who was guiding him to face an unkind world that judged him long time before even having sexual desires or having his first sexual experience. Despite being guided how to intelligently respond to those attacks, being targeted impacted his confidence, self-esteem, and self-worth; he often felt sick and refused to continue going to kindergarten.

If that was not enough, the bullying continued in primary school, despite his schoolteacher trying to tell other children in the class to accept his "effeminate side." Despite her meaning well, he felt even more hurt and stopped talking to anyone about what was going on in his inner world. The bullying continued in middle and high school and at the oratory summer camps, and the insults became even greater. As a result, he had very few male friends, was marginalized, and always counted on female friends to make him feel good enough and worthy.

Throughout his early years, his mental and emotional well-being were severely impacted by judgments, prejudice, and religious views on sexuality. He perceived the people around him were convinced he was a "pervert" not worthy of anything. The feelings of shame and guilt arousing from judgments of others forced him to isolate and protect himself. He would hide anything that some people would perceive as effeminate from himself and anyone who would come near him. He focused all his energy into studying and used learning to play piano and singing as an outlet to release the built-up pressure from all those violent emotions and intentions.

At sixteen, because of his lung collapsing, he was hospitalized; it is during this time that his love for medicine started. He decided, in helping others, he will be more accepted in society and redeem himself by displaying "saintly" behaviors. The way his surgeons treated him made him feel dehumanized, and all the issues he faced there inspired him further to pursue medicine so he can make a difference and bring the so-needed changes that everyone could benefit from.

Having spent all his youth in a town where he did not feel accepted, loved, and appreciated for who he was, he was drawn toward more cosmopolitan cities, intelligent open-minded people, so he welcomed with open arms the opportunity to go to university in Milan.

By then, it was clear to Pietro that trying to suffocate an important part of him not only did not work, but also, it was toxic; "praying the gay away" or living in denial only exacerbated feelings of worthlessness, loneliness, and despair. Back then, there were no positive role models about being homosexual; he grew up at the time of the AIDS crisis, and the only examples of gay people in the media were either those made fun of in movies and TV shows or those dying alone and rejected by their families. Nevertheless, logic, intuition, and a strong survival instinct guided him as he could no longer believe there was no other way; he started to search for people who were going through the same.

At some point, in Duomo Square in Milan, he summoned the courage to go to a newsagent and pick up a magazine to understand his feelings and learn more about being gay in non-shameful, nonjudgmental, and more accepting ways. He learned there was a gay book library, a gay association, a community of progressive people, gay bars, etc. He started to quench his thirst of nineteen years of suffering, isolation, and shame. His concern about the well-being of other gay people made him join gay activism against homophobia and bullying.

He got a master's degree in medicine and surgery, Summa cum Laude, at the University of Milan, discussing a dissertation on heart rate variability.

Having witnessed how nepotism, servility, and corruption heavily impacted upon doctors' careers and the running of healthcare, he preferred to make uncomfortable choices rather than getting involved in any of that. Having found no opportunities to get into specialty training near home, he moved to Florence for his specialty studies. He specialized in acute internal medicine at the University of Florence with an MSc dissertation on pulmonary embolism.

Perceiving no fair career opportunities in his home country and wanting to avoid becoming as frustrated as many colleagues he had met during his studies, he started looking for alternative paths. After a period of research and reflection, he chose to relocate to London, UK, and pursue a career in acute medicine.

He started familiarizing with the new work environment with an honorary contract as clinical and research fellow while joining the Society for Acute Medicine and continuing his medical studies, attaining Collegiate Membership of the Royal College of Physicians.

A solid "old-fashioned" academic foundation combined with ambition and a caring attitude toward patients and fellow healthcare workers worked as fuel for his subsequent career.

He joined the acute medicine training program as an opportunity to gain an extensive work experience in different hospital settings and several clinical specialties, completed the Specialty Certificate Examination in acute medicine and progressed in the medical career from junior registrar up to consultant and clinical director.

His personal journey overcoming cultural and religious prejudice forged an inquisitive mind always questioning the status quo and unwilling to being subdued. To overcome his emotional battles made him seek ways to learn, grow, and find solutions to the causes of pain and suffering.

Combining his Italian directness, humor, and warmth with attention to detail, drive for quality, and desire to help others and solve problems, Dr. Pietro did not hold back joining or launching working groups and initiatives for patient safety, quality improvement, and service development. Having a broad range of experience in different settings also helps him notice and question details that others become blind to because of habit and familiarity.

Having experienced great mentors and teachers, his desire to contribute to supporting and mentoring younger doctors grew him into an educator who initiated and delivered teaching initiatives in bedside ultrasonography.

A keen and open-minded learner, he continues to broaden his skill set in the conventional medical field, attending courses, conferences, congresses and keeping up to date with the relevant literature. His quest in finding solutions for patients' and personal health challenges and to promote and restore comprehensive health and well-being brought him to also explore other disciplines.

He experienced the benefits of complementary and integrative methods, such as osteopathy, ayurveda, acupuncture, herbal medicine, biodynamic therapy, etc. His interest in nutrition, health promotion, and healthy aging brought him to attend several conferences of integrative medicine and professional courses in functional medicine, which have also provided him with opportunities to visit international hospitals and health centers.

His spiritual journey includes qualifying as accredited BAHA Healer at the School of Intuition and Healing, training in Neo-Tantra, practicing yoga and meditation. His personal development journey included training with Landmark Education.

He joined the European Institute of Innovation and Technology – Health KIC Advanced Management Programme on Health Innovation run by Imperial College London, IESE Business School, and Copenhagen Business School to learn from and connect with innovators who share a similar call for healthcare improvement. He welcomed the opportunity to learn about other countries' healthcare systems, visit innovative hospitals, health tech companies and start-ups, and network with like-minded individuals.

Over the last six years, he has embarked on a profound journey of self-reflection, learning, and transformation with world-renowned human behavior, cognition, and emotional intelligence expert Tony J. Selimi to bring clarity of intention in his life, maximize his human potential, and use all his wisdom to empower other doctors and Purposefully Transforming Healthcare®.

Besides providing clinical care as acute physician, clinical and educational supervision to doctors in training as consultant and medical leadership as clinical director, he founded Transforming Healthcare Ltd with a vision to contribute toward assisting doctors and everyone involved in healthcare to create sustainable solutions for thriving environments.

His mission is realized though publishing books, writing articles, delivering talks, interviews, consultations, training, and partnering with and influencing world leaders, healthcare stakeholders, and policymakers.

He believes that health is priceless, and therefore, healthcare is always worthy of investing in. He believes that everyone is worthy of love and of full expression of their human potential. Dr. Pietro knows that doctors and everyone else in healthcare benefit from having a nurturing environment to provide high-quality care consistently. He loves to create innovative solutions that relieve frustrations currently affecting patients and healthcare providers. He has an unshakeable trust that doctors, healthcare providers, and healthcare stakeholders can develop mutually beneficial relationships based on clear aligned goals. He trusts how Purposefully Transforming Healthcare® can reawaken lost enthusiasm and love for the medical profession.

In transforming beliefs that create prejudice, lack of dialogue, and lack of resources, funding can be made available to providing scientific evidence for the benefit of complementary healing modalities to be integrated into modern medicine. It is what can shift us from the current medical paradigm which treats the symptoms and the effects of some illness by interfering with the mechanisms of disease toward an innovative way of addressing the root causes of disease.

His research articles appeared on the *American Journal of Medicine, Circulation,* and *BMJ Quality Improvement Reports.* He spoke at the Mediterranean Emergency Medicine Congress and the Care Bundles Conference. The achievements of the Ambulatory Emergency Care Unit appeared in the *Ambulatory Emergency Care Network Newsletter.* His contribution to gay activism included speaking about bullying and homophobia in high schools in Italy, holding workshops at neo-Tantra festivals, and liaising with sexual health services stakeholders.

Dr. Pietro's wide-ranging experience gives him a broader understanding of the challenges that medicine as a profession and an industry faces. His vision and mission are to be the beacon of light for other doctors to work in partnership and in synergy with decision-makers to purposefully transform healthcare, creating a thriving environment, providing high-quality care. He leaves colleagues feeling heard, empowered, and inspired to be part of a valued profession.

ACKNOWLEDGMENTS

"No man is an island" is a phrase from a famous poem by John Donne that makes us realize how we all depend and rely on one another.

Listing everyone who has had an impact upon me and consequently on the writing and content of this book is an arduous and, frankly, impossible task; every interaction with another human being has taught me something about who I am, what I am here to do, and why do I do what I do. The more I learned to self-reflect, the more I was able to track the origins of my thoughts, beliefs, ideas, and authentic values I hold dear to my heart. In acknowledging something that has happened in my past, I am now able to share transformational insights to help fellow doctors and others involved in providing healthcare feel acknowledged and valued. Even those interactions that, at the time, I perceived as negative and painful contributed to what I am today and continue to evolve for the rest of my life.

Specifically, a lot of topics and ideas contained in this book were born as a result of many hours of suffering, struggle, confrontation, moaning, despair, and anger that challenged me at the core. It is a way to use all that crushed me to develop an attitude of gratitude. In retrospect, in overcoming those frustrations and problems, I was inspired to write and develop useful solutions for others.

My sincere heartfelt gratitude goes toward all the teachers, students, professors, supervisors, supervisees, mentors, mentees, colleagues, coworkers, employers, contractors, friends, acquaintances, family, relatives, school mates, partners, lovers, haters, doctors, patients, and everyone else who contributed to a lifetime of learning through support and challenge, which has contributed to who I am today. Thank you!

Having said that, a special thank-you goes to my loving parents, Egidio and Mariagrazia, who, after giving me life, supported and challenged me in a nurturing way throughout my life. Thank you from the bottom of my heart for everything! Furthermore, a big thank-you goes to my loving sister, Daniela, and her family for their love, kindness, and support.

To all the teachers at school, thank you for patiently educating me. I have been blessed with some great professors at university. Thank you for sharing your knowledge with me. I am grateful to all mentors, tutors, supervisors, and colleagues for teaching me how to be a doctor. To all the educators, presenters, speakers, organizers of the numerous courses, conferences, and workshops I participated to over the years, thank you for supporting my continuous growth. To all the employers, managers, coworkers, colleagues in several workplaces, thank you for your support and challenge and for believing in me.

A special thank-you goes to Tony J. Selimi, without whom this book would not have been possible. Thank you for relentlessly believing in me, lovingly challenging me when my fears and doubts prevailed, supporting me in carrying out the hard work, daring to aspire to bigger things, and broadening my horizon. Seeing this book take shape as a result of all those efforts fills my heart with gratitude and love.

My deep gratitude goes to you, the reader, and to my dear friends who volunteered to be the first ones to read this inspired book, share openheartedly their feedback, and write a testimonial and an introduction. Reading your reactions and appreciation filled my heart with joy and reassured me that this book and pursuing my vision to purposefully transform healthcare can truly make a difference.

And finally, a special thank you goes to my soul, for enduring the pain and intuitively guiding and supporting me on my ever-evolving vision, mission, and purpose in life.

NOTES

Printed in the United States
by Baker & Taylor Publisher Services